Secrets of
LIVING
FAT-FREE

Hints, tips, recipes, and strategies for losing weight and feeling great

SANDRA WOODRUFF, RD

Avery Publishing Group
Garden City Park, New York

Front Cover Photograph: Comstock
Cover design: William Gonzalez
Typesetting: William Gonzalez
In-House Editor: Joanne Abrams

Avery Publishing Group
120 Old Broadway
Garden City Park, NY 11040
1-800-548-5757

Library of Congress Cataloging-in-Publication-Data

Woodruff, Sandra L.
    Secrets of Living Fat-Free: hints, tips, recipes, and strategies
for losing weight and feeling great / Sandra Woodruff.
        p. cm.
    Includes index.
    ISBN 0-89529-787-6

    1. Low-fat diet. 2. Low-fat diet—Recipes. I. Title.
RM237.7.W665 1997
641.5′638—dc21   97-6065
                                                          CIP

Printed in the United States of America

10 9 8 7 6 5

Contents

This book is dedicated to my favorite
taste testers, Wiley and C.D.

Acknowledgments

I t has been a great pleasure to produce this book with the talented and dedicated professionals at Avery Publishing Group, who have so generously lent their support and creativity at every stage of production. Special thanks go to Rudy Shur and Ken Rajman for providing the opportunity to publish this book, and to my editor, Joanne Abrams, whose hard work, endless patience, and diligent attention to detail have added so much.

Thanks also go to my dear friends and family members for their enduring support and encouragement, and to my clients and coworkers, whose questions and ideas keep me learning and experimenting with new things. Last, but not least, I would like to thank my husband, Tom Maureau, for his long-term support and encouragement, and for always being there for me.

Preface

No one can dispute the benefits of eating a low-fat diet. Everyone knows that a low-fat diet is one of the keys to successful weight control. A healthful diet makes it easier to both lose unwanted pounds and *keep* them off. Just as important, diets that are low in fat and high in wholesome, nutrient-rich foods have been linked with a reduced risk of cancer, heart disease, and many other illnesses. They improve your overall health, they boost your energy, and they enhance your feelings of well-being. As a result, people have become increasingly fat-conscious, and counting fat grams has become a national pastime. Food manufacturers, restaurateurs, and other merchants have responded with a multitude of excellent new products, and eating healthfully has never been easier or more enjoyable.

Despite this new fat-consciousness, many people are daunted by the task of getting the fat out of their diet. They simply don't know where to start. From shopping for groceries and preparing home-cooked meals to dining out, fat seems to be a part of life. How do you know which are the best choices? Unless you're a nutrition expert, it's hard to be sure. And the wealth of new products and deluge of often-contradictory information seems to add to the confusion. This is why *Secrets of Living Fat-Free* was written.

In Chapter 1, *Secrets of Living Fat-Free* begins by explaining—in understandable terms—what you should know about the different kinds of fats in foods, and by providing you with plenty of reasons to get the fat out of your life. Chapter 2 then teaches you how to budget your own daily fat intake, and how, by following a few simple guidelines, you can not only stick to your fat budget, but also improve the overall quality of your diet. Included in this practical chapter are some simple steps that will allow you to lose weight through healthy dietary and lifestyle changes.

Chapters 3 and 4 will guide you in buying the best low- and no-fat products available. First, Chapter 3 teaches you how to interpret a food label, and how to use that label to quickly discriminate between a food that will help you meet your dietary goals, and a food that you want to avoid. Chapter 4 then provides all the supermarket strategies you'll need to get the fat out of your shopping cart and replace it with healthy, satisfying low-fat foods.

To be sure that you can use your pantry of fat-free foods to make delicious low-fat and fat-free dishes, Chapter 5 provides a wealth of fat-free cooking tips. Then Chapter 6 presents a collection of tantalizing fat-free recipes—recipes designed to provide minimum fat, and maximum taste and nutrition.

Find it hardest to fight fat when you're away from home? Chapter 7 shares secrets of low-fat living that will help you in many everyday and special activities, from traveling on a plane, to grabbing a snack at the office, to enjoying a holiday party, to dining at your favorite Mexican restaurant. This chapter will prove to you that you don't have to sacrifice your social life or any of your usual pleasures or pursuits to get the fat out of your life.

Finally, in Chapter 8, you will discover how exercise can be an effective "secret" weapon in the fight against fat.

Through your choices, you have tremendous power to determine your health and the quality of your life. The information presented in this book will help you make the best choices possible. Organized for easy access, this practical guide makes it a snap to find the information you want, when you want it. It is my hope that *Secrets of Living Fat-Free* will become a reference that you turn to time and time again, and that will show you that fat-free living is possible every day of the year.

Introduction

E ating great food is one of life's simplest yet greatest pleasures. And there is nothing wrong with enjoying good food—except that for too long, *good* often meant *greasy*. Butter, margarine, oil, mayonnaise, cheese, highly-marbled meats, and other rich foods were long considered an essential part of good eating. We now know that all this fat—along with excess sugar and salt—has a tremendous impact on the way we look and feel. First, it has been well established that high-fat diets have been a chief contributor to the expanding national waistline. Moreover, diseases like obesity, cancer, and diabetes have all been found to be directly related to high-fat, nutrient-poor diets, and to greatly affect the quality of life for millions of Americans. The good news is that just as certain foods can detract from health, other foods can promote vibrant health, weight loss, and longevity.

As a nutritionist who has been helping people modify their eating habits for well over a decade, I have witnessed firsthand the profound changes that occur after people get the fat out of their diets—greater success in losing and maintaining weight, dramatic drops in blood cholesterol and triglycerides, reduced blood pressure and body fat, and greatly enhanced energy levels and feelings of well-being. When this happens, people are quite often surprised. Why? They simply can't believe that they did not have to suffer, feel deprived, or starve themselves to bring about these improvements. They also can't believe how easy it is to maintain their low-fat lifestyles in a vast array of situations, for never before has there been such a great selection of low-fat foods—so many ways to eat both well *and* wisely.

Secrets of Living Fat-Free was written to help you use the power of food to reap the same benefits enjoyed by my clients. This easy-to-use, practical reference will guide you in making the best food choices possible—wherever you go, whatever you do. From making a home-cooked meal to going out on the town, you will find that there are plenty of delicious options for maintaining a fat-free lifestyle. But unlike many books about fat-free eating, *Secrets of Living Fat-Free* goes beyond fat, because if you want optimal health, you also need optimal nutrition. As you will see, just because a food is low-fat or fat-free, it is not necessarily good for you. The array of nutrient-poor, sugar-laden fat-free foods that has entered the marketplace has created a whole new set of

1

problems for the unaware consumer, including—believe it or not!—weight gain. *Secrets of Living Fat-Free* alerts you to these problems, and shows you how to balance your diet. It helps you avoid the common pitfalls of fat-free eating, and become trimmer, healthier, and more vital.

Within these pages, you will discover that watching your fat intake and eating healthfully does not have to mean dieting and deprivation. This book is filled with easy-to-follow guidelines, helpful hints, fat-saving tips, and tricks of the trade that will help you and every member of your family say good-bye to all that excess fat. I wish you the best of luck and health in all your fat-free eating adventures!

1. A Short Course in Fats

During the past few years, fat-free eating has increasingly become a topic of great interest. Why? The health benefits of reducing dietary fat are becoming more and more obvious each day. From excess weight, to heart disease, to cancer, to diabetes, and more, a long list of preventable health problems has been undeniably linked to excess dietary fat. Low-fat living, on the other hand, has been undeniably linked with increased success in losing and maintaining weight, and with greater vibrance and health.

Though more and more people are now aware of the need to get the fat out of their diets, many people simply don't know where to start. Between the abundance of new products that are constantly entering the market, the confusing advertising claims made about fat-free and low-fat products, and the often-contradictory information presented in the media, changing over to a low-fat lifestyle can be a daunting task. How do you know how much fat you should be eating every day? And how do you choose the foods that will keep your fat intake within these limits? Furthermore, are some fats more healthful than others—and is it possible to eat too *little* fat? *Secrets of Living Fat-Free* was written to answer these questions and many more. Within the pages of this book, you will also discover the secrets of selecting the best low- and no-fat foods at the grocery store, as well as how to get the fat out of your favorite family recipes. You will also learn how to spot unwanted fats in every situation imaginable—from dining out in your favorite restaurant to grabbing a snack on the run—and how to make healthy, satisfying choices each and every time.

This chapter will explain some basic facts that everyone should know about fat. You will learn about the different kinds of fats in foods, and will discover which fats are needed in your diet, and which should be avoided. The rest of the chapter will explain just how fat affects your health, and will provide you with plenty of reasons to learn the secrets of fat-free living.

WHAT YOU SHOULD KNOW ABOUT FAT

Fat is a nutrient, and like all nutrients, some fat is essential for life. However, there are many kinds of fats, and while some contribute to good health, others can con-

3

tribute to a myriad of problems, ranging from cancer to heart disease to arthritis. And, of course, too much of *any* kind of fat can lead to obesity. In this section, you will learn why you do need some fat, and you will discover which fats are beneficial, and which have no place in a healthful lifestyle.

Why You Need Fat

Fat performs a variety of vital functions in the body. Fat forms a part of the membrane that surrounds every cell of the body, allowing fat-soluble vitamins, hormones, and other substances to enter and leave as needed. Small fat pads located throughout the body act like shock absorbers for the organs. Fat also forms a layer beneath the skin, insulating the body from temperature extremes. Like carbohydrates, fat is an essential fuel that is burned for energy by muscle cells and many other cells of the body. And, as many people know too well, fat is deposited in fat cells as a way of storing excess calories when the amount of food eaten exceeds the amount that can be burned for energy.

Just as fat is important in the body, it is an important part of the diet. Dietary fat aids in the absorption of fat-soluble nutrients like vitamins A, D, E, and K from the digestive tract into the blood. Once these nutrients are absorbed, fat also facilitates their transport throughout the body. Certain kinds of dietary fats—known as essential fatty acids—also function as essential nutrients. These fats help maintain healthy skin and hair, and are involved in a wide variety of body processes.

Despite all of fat's important functions, we need only a small amount in our daily diets. Moreover, as many people know, an excess can be disastrous. In addition, not all fats are equal in terms of their healthfulness. Let's take a look at the different kinds of dietary fats, so that you can be sure to get enough of the ones you need while avoiding the ones that you don't need.

Types of Fat

Basically, there are three main classes of dietary fats: saturated, monounsaturated, and polyunsaturated. These terms all refer to the degree to which a fat molecule is loaded with hydrogen atoms. Saturated fats, for instance, are fully loaded with hydrogen, while polyunsaturated fats contain the fewest hydrogen atoms.

Two more types of fat also have a bearing on your health. One, cholesterol, has received a lot of attention for many years. The other, trans-fatty acids, were more recently identified.

When looking at the different fats contained in a given food, it's important to realize that any one food generally contains a mixture of these fats, rather than just one type. Nevertheless, many foods are much higher in one type than another, which is why a food may be referred to as being "polyunsaturated" or "monounsaturated."

Saturated Fat

Saturated fat—so named because it is fully saturated with hydrogen atoms—is best known for its role in promoting heart disease. This fat encourages the development of heart disease by raising blood cholesterol levels, and thus leading to clogged arteries.

How do you know if a fat is saturated? Since these fats are solid at room temperature, it is often quite obvious. For example, the fat around a piece of beef or pork is solid because it contains a high proportion of saturated fat. Chicken fat, which is lower in saturated fat, is somewhat softer. A stick of butter is also solid because it is rich in saturated fat. And since full-fat dairy products like whole milk, cream, and whole milk cheeses contain butterfat, they are also high in saturated fats.

Saturated fats are also abundant in tropical oils like coconut and palm oil, which are sometimes used in baked goods like cookies and crackers, and in other processed foods. However, most processed foods these days are made with partially *hydrogenated* vegetable oils—chemically altered fats made by adding hydrogen to liquid vegetable oils. Why do this? Adding hydrogenation to liquid oils transforms them into solid margarines and shortenings. But while hydrogenation improves the cooking and baking qualities of oils, and extends their shelf life as well, it makes the oils more saturated and also creates undesirable by-products known as *trans-fatty acids*, or *trans fats*. Unfortunately, trans fats act much like saturated fats to raise blood cholesterol levels. Many researchers believe that trans fats may be linked to some forms of cancer, and to other health problems, as well.

Monounsaturated Fat

Unlike saturated fats, monounsaturated fats like olive oil and canola oil do not promote heart disease. In fact, in countries like Greece and Italy, where close to 40 percent of the calories in the average diet come from olive oil, the incidence of heart disease is much lower than it is in countries like the United States. Does this mean that olive oil is *good* for you? No. People in these countries eat olive oil *instead* of saturated fats. It is the absence of saturated fat, rather than the presence of monounsaturated fat, that provides the health benefits. However, since monounsaturated fats have no known harmful effects—other than being a concentrated source of calories, like all fats—they are a good fat choice as long as you stay within your fat budget. Other foods rich in monounsaturated fat include peanuts, peanut oil, avocados, almonds, cashews, and macadamia nuts.

Polyunsaturated Fat

Like monounsaturated fats, polyunsaturated fats do not raise blood cholesterol levels, so they are often recommended as part of a heart-healthy diet. In addition, certain polyunsaturated fats are essential for life, and must be included in our diets. The first of these essential fats, *linoleic acid*, belongs to a family of fats known as the omega-6 fatty acids, and is naturally abundant in nuts and seeds. The average adult needs at least 3 to 6 grams of linoleic acid per day—the amount present in about two teaspoonfuls of polyunsaturated vegetable oil (such as corn, safflower, and sunflower) or about two tablespoonfuls of nuts or seeds (such as walnuts or sunflower seeds). The second kind of essential fat, *linolenic acid*, belongs to the omega-3 family of fatty acids. While this fat is present mainly in fish and leafy green vegetables, flax seeds are another rich source, and walnuts and soy products provide some linolenic acid, as well. No formal recommendation regarding linolenic acid intake exists in the United States, but researchers believe that we need about a quarter as much linolenic acid as we do linoleic acid. The Canadian government recommends a minimum of 1.1 grams of linolenic acid per day for adult women and 1.5 grams for adult men.

Omega-6 and omega-3 fats are important because they are the raw materials for *eicosanoids*—hormone-like substances that control many aspects of metabolism, including blood clotting, blood pressure regulation, inflammation, and immune system function. There is still much to be learned about omega-6 and omega-3 fatty acids, but many researchers believe that humans evolved on a diet that provided about equal amounts of these fats. This began to change rapidly around the turn of the century, when industry developed ways to mass produce vegetable oils rich in omega-6

Getting the Right Balance of Essential Fats

Two kinds of essential fats are needed in the diet every day. The first is an omega-6 fat known as linoleic acid, and the other is an omega-3 fat known as linolenic acid. Most people eat far too much omega-6 fat and too little omega-3 fat—and the health implications of doing so include an increased risk of blood clots, high blood pressure, cancer, and various inflammatory diseases. Most foods provide a mixture of these two fats, and a food is usually higher in one type of fatty acid than it is in another. Clearly, it makes sense to choose foods that provide the most healthy balance of these fats.

The following table lists the omega-6 and omega-3 content of selected foods, along with the ratio of omega-6 to omega-3 fats. When evaluating this table, keep two things in mind. First, we need only small amounts of these fats in our diets. About 3 to 6 grams of linoleic acid and 1.1 to 1.5 grams of linolenic acid are the minimum suggested amounts. Second, the balance or ratio of these two fats in your diet is just as important as the amounts. Most Americans eat at least ten times as much omega-6 fats as they do omega-3 fats. Researchers estimate that some people may be eating up to *twenty times* more omega-6 fats than omega-3 fats. And while no one is sure exactly what the optimal ratio is, it is thought that a diet that provides only four to six times as much omega-6 as omega-3 would greatly reduce the risk of many diseases.

By examining this table, you will see how foods like vegetables, fruits, and fish contribute to a favorable balance of fats. You will also notice that meats like venison have the most favorable ratio of omega-6 to omega-3 fats. Why? Wild game feeds mostly on green plants, which provide them with omega-3 fats. On the other hand, domestic livestock consumes more grains, which make their meat higher not only in total fat, but also in omega-6 fats. This table also makes it easy to see how liberal use of foods like corn oil, sunflower oil, and safflower oil—and fats. At the same time, farmers began feeding their livestock grains, which made the animals fatter—and higher in omega-6 fats. As people began eating more fatty meats, as well as more vegetable oils—in fried foods, salad dressings, mayonnaise, margarine, and baked goods—the ratio of omega-6 to omega-3 fats in the diet rose from about 1 to 1 to as high as 20 to 1. And while the eicosanoids made from omega-6 fats are vital—they enable blood to clot, maintain normal blood pressure and immune function, and perform many other essential functions—when omega-6 fats are consumed in excess, the resulting overabundance of eicosanoids favors the development of blood clots, high blood pressure, cancerous tumors, and inflammatory diseases.

At the same time that many people are overdosing on omega-6 fat, they are getting too little omega-3 fat. Why? Most people eat very little fish and not nearly

related products like full-fat margarine, mayonnaise, and salad dressings—are major contributors to an omega-6 overdose.

Don't get too caught up trying to calculate your ratio of omega-6 to omega-3 fats. If you follow the Guidelines for Good Eating, presented on page 21, you will automatically consume a healthful balance of these essential nutrients.

Essential Fatty Acid Content of Selected Foods

Food	Omega-6 Fats	Omega-3 Fats	Omega-6 to Omega-3 Ratio
Spinach, raw (2 cups)	0.02 g	0.13 g	0.2 to 1
Salmon, poached (4 ounces)	0.49 g	1.78 g	0.3 to 1
Flax seeds (2 tbsp)*	1.06 g	3.23 g	0.3 to 1
Strawberries (2 cups)	0.36 g	0.26 g	1.4 to 1
Canola oil (1 tbsp)	2.77 g	1.27 g	2.2 to 1
Walnuts (2 tbsp)	4.8 g	1.02 g	4.7 to 1
Venison, roasted (4 ounces)	0.6 g	0.1 g	6.0 to 1
Soybean oil (1 tbsp)	6.95 g	0.93 g	7.5 to 1
Tofu (4 ounces)	2.7 g	0.36 g	7.5 to 1
Skinless chicken breast, roasted (4 ounces)	0.74 g	0.07 g	10.6 to 1
Olive oil (1 tbsp)	1.07 g	0.08 g	13.3 to 1
Beef rib eye steak, broiled and trimmed (4 ounces)	0.35 g	0.02 g	17.5 to 1
Corn oil (1 tbsp)	7.9 g	0.10 g	79 to 1
Sunflower oil (1 tbsp)	8.95 g	0.05 g	179 to 1
Safflower oil (1 tbsp)	10.1 g	0.05 g	202 to 1

*For information about flax seeds, see the inset "Flax Facts" on page 8.

Flax Facts

Want to know a great way to add health-promoting omega-3 fatty acids to your diet? Try tossing flax seeds into your dishes. Small and nutty-tasting, flax seeds are available in health foods stores. They are very economical, and can be stored at room temperature for several months. Best of all, they can be used in a surprising number of ways.

Probably the easiest way to enjoy the goodness of flax is to sprinkle the seeds on hot or cold cereal. Or try adding them to breads, muffins, and other baked goods. Flax seeds can also be ground into meal using a blender or food processor. The resulting product, which looks similar to wheat bran, can be sprinkled over cereal, just like the whole seeds. It can also be substituted for up to a quarter of the flour in baked goods. The slightly sweet, nutty taste of flax enhances the flavors of muffins, breads, and other goods. And flax meal is a natural in low-fat and fat-free baking. Because it contains fibers and gums, the meal will improve the texture of your reduced-fat products. Just keep in mind that once ground into meal, the seeds can turn rancid quickly, so try to prepare the meal just before use. When you do have leftovers, store the meal in an opaque container in the refrigerator, and use it within a week.

Looking for a great egg substitute for baked goods? Place 1 1/2 tablespoons of flax seeds in a mini-blender jar, and blend until finely ground. Then add 1/4 cup plus 2 tablespoons of water, and blend for another minute, or until the mixture thickens to the consistency of raw egg whites. Use 3 tablespoons of this mixture to replace 1 whole egg, or use 2 tablespoons to replace 1 egg white. Like flax meal, this mixture should be made fresh for each use.

---

enough vegetables. Another problem is that omega-6 fat competes with omega-3 fat for processing by the body. So when people eat large amounts of omega-6 fat, it blocks the metabolism of what little omega-3 fat they do eat, making matters worse. Why do we need omega-3 fats? Like omega-6 fats, omega-3 fats are made into eicosanoids, but omega-3 eicosanoids alter body chemistry in a very different way. They "thin" the blood, thereby preventing deadly blood clots from forming. They also help to lower blood pressure, reduce blood triglycerides, inhibit tumor formation, and protect against inflammatory diseases like rheumatoid arthritis.

It has become obvious that too much omega-6 fat and too little omega-3 fat plays an important role in promoting a number of diseases. How can you restore the right balance of fat to your diet? Reduce the amount of omega-6 fat in your diet to a healthy level by minimizing the use of vegetable oils, shortenings, full-fat margarine, full-fat mayonnaise, and fatty meats. Instead, eat a diet rich in vegetables, fruits, and whole grains, with fish several times a week, small amounts of nuts and seeds, and, if desired, lean meats. The inset "Getting the Right Balance of Essential Fats," found on page 6, provides more information on omega-6 and omega-3 fats.

Cholesterol

This fatty substance helps form the protective sheaths that surround nerve fibers; is the raw material for the body's production of vitamin D and many other hormones; and is an important component of all cell membranes. Despite this, the dietary requirement for cholesterol is zero—your body can make all the cholesterol it needs. And eating too much cholesterol can raise blood cholesterol levels beyond healthy levels, contributing to clogged arteries.

Which foods are high in cholesterol? Cholesterol is found only in animal products, so that meats, dairy products, and eggs (the yolks only) are all sources. Do lean meats contain less cholesterol than fatty meats? No. Because cholesterol is a component of muscle cells, lean meats contain just as much cholesterol as their fatty counterparts. However, since saturated fats, found in fatty meats, raise blood cholesterol levels even more than dietary cholesterol does, lean meats are, of course, the better choice. As for dairy products, the low-fat versions have significantly less cholesterol than the full-fat versions, and fat-free dairy products are practically cholesterol-free. If you limit meats, poultry, and seafood to six ounces or less per day, limit egg yolks to four per week, and choose nonfat dairy products, you can keep your cholesterol intake below the recommended upper limit of 300 milligrams per day.

It is important to be aware that the recommendation for cholesterol—and for fat, as well—does not apply to infants and children under the age of two, as they *do* need cholesterol for their developing brain and nervous system. Breast milk, the preferred food for infants, is rich in both cholesterol and fat for this very reason. (For information on blood cholesterol, see the inset "Understanding Your Blood Cholesterol Level" on page 12.)

LOW-FAT LIVING—YOUR LIFE DEPENDS ON IT

You have just learned about the different kinds of dietary fats, and have discovered which fats contribute to good health, and which fats should be avoided. People who eat diets rich in whole, natural foods such as vegetables, fruits, and whole grains; include fish in their diet several times a week; and enjoy small amounts of nuts and seeds will have no problem getting the right amount and balance of essential fats. Most people, though, consume *excess* dietary fat, and too much saturated fat, in particular. In fact, diet is the number-two cause of preventable death in Americans (smoking is number one), and too much fat is the main contributing factor. This section describes the role that excess fat and other dietary factors play in promoting disease, and provides plenty of reasons to learn the secrets of fat-free living.

Diet—A Key to Weight Control

There are plenty of good reasons to fight fat, but perhaps the most common one is the desire to lose weight. How does fighting fat help with weight loss? With more than twice the calories of carbohydrates or protein, fat is a concentrated source of calories. Compare the calorie count of a cup of butter or margarine (almost pure fat) with that of a cup of flour (almost pure carbohydrates). The butter has 1,600 calories, and the

The Facts About Fake Fats

How do manufacturers get the fat out of fat-free and low-fat foods? A variety of substitutes are used. The most commonly used fat substitutes are made from carbohydrates. Among these are vegetable gums, such as guar and xanthan gums; and modified food starches, made from potatoes, cornstarch, rice, oats, or tapioca. These products are generally combined with water to add thickness to and retain moisture in a variety of fat-free and low-fat foods, from salad dressings, mayonnaise, and margarine, to baked goods. Many baked goods also use fruit purées and a variety of plant fibers to add and hold in moisture when the fat is eliminated. These carbohydrate-based fat substitutes are very safe, and greatly reduce the fat and calories in many fat-free and low-fat products.

Protein-based fat substitutes such as nonfat milk solids, whey protein concentrate, and soy protein are also used in a variety of nonfat and low-fat products—including baked goods and nonfat ice cream—where they provide structure, creaminess, and thickness. For instance, the fat substitute Simplesse, which is used in some nonfat frozen desserts, is made from milk and egg white proteins. Since protein-based fat substitutes like Simplesse provide about half as many calories as the fat they replace, you do not get the same type of calorie savings when using these products as you get with carbohydrate-based fat substitutes made from plant fibers and vegetable gums. These carbohydrate-based substitutes provide almost no calories, and allow more water to be incorporated into the product. (Carbohydrate-based fat substitutes made from food starches and corn syrup provide more calories—about 4 per gram.)

The most controversial fat substitute is olestra. A synthetic combination of sucrose (sugar) and fatty acids, olestra cannot be absorbed by the body, and so provides no calories at all. Unlike other fat substitutes, olestra can be used for frying, and is being incorporated into fat-free snack foods like potato chips. But while olestra imparts the flavor and feel of fat to foods, it is not without problems. You see, olestra binds with fat-soluble nutrients like vitamins A, D, E, and K; with the carotenoids, such as beta-carotene; and perhaps with other nutrients not yet identified. It then carries them out of the body. Because olestra causes the malabsorption of nutrients, it is fortified with vitamins A, D, E, and K—but not with carotenoids or any other nutrients. Many researchers fear that eating olestra products will cause blood levels of carotenoids to become dangerously low, setting the stage for cancer, heart disease, and other health problems. If that's not enough to worry about, olestra also causes abdominal cramping and diarrhea in some people.

The best policy is to stick with foods that use carbohydrate-based fat substitutes, such as vegetable gums, food starches, fruit purées, and plant fibers. Also, look for foods whose fat has been eliminated by a change of cooking methods—by baking instead of frying, for instance.

Understanding Blood Pressure

What is blood pressure? It is the measurement of the force exerted by the blood on the wall of your blood vessels. Two numbers are used to measure this force. The top number, or systolic blood pressure, is the pressure inside the arteries when the heart contracts. The bottom number, or diastolic blood pressure, is the pressure inside the arteries when the heart relaxes between beats. A normal blood pressure reading is considered to be around 120/80. When these numbers reach 140/90, a person is considered to have high blood pressure, or hypertension.

One in six Americans has high blood pressure—over 40 million people in all. Many are not even aware of it. What does this mean in terms of health risks? Because the heart must work harder to pump the blood through the cardiovascular system of a hypertensive person, even slightly elevated blood pressure can increase the risk of heart attack and stroke.

What can you do about high blood pressure? Plenty. First and foremost, adopt a low-fat, low-salt diet that includes plenty of vegetables, fruits, legumes, and whole grains. The tips presented in this book will show you how to do just that without sacrificing flavor or satisfaction. If necessary, control calories to allow for gradual weight loss. Losing just ten pounds can significantly reduce blood pressure in many people. Exercise regularly. This will not only keep your cardiovascular system strong and assist with weight control, but will also help you deal with stress, a potent contributor to high blood pressure. And, of course, don't smoke, and don't drink alcohol in excess. Together, these simple measures are so powerful that they can eliminate the need for medication in many people.

flour has 400 calories. It's easy to see where most of our calories come from.

Besides being high in calories, fat is also readily converted into body fat when eaten in excess. Carbohydrate-rich foods eaten in excess are also stored as body fat, but they must first be converted into fat—a process that burns up some of the carbohydrates. The bottom line is that a high-fat diet will cause 20 percent more weight gain than will a high-carbohydrate diet, even when the two diets contain the same number of calories. So a high-fat diet is a double-edged sword for the weight-conscious person. It is high in calories, and it is the kind of nutrient that is most readily stored as body fat.

Does changing to a low-fat diet guarantee weight loss? Unfortunately, no. As will be explained in Chapter 2, not *all* low-fat foods are also low in calories. But when chosen wisely, low-fat and fat-free foods can help you reach and maintain a healthy body weight. (See the inset "Simple Steps to Successful Weight Loss" on page 19 for tried-and-true weight-loss strategies.)

Diet and Cardiovascular Disorders

The link between diet and cardiovascular disease—which continues to be the number-

---

Understanding Your Blood Cholesterol Level

A high blood cholesterol level is a strong risk factor for heart disease. Fortunately, by following the guidelines presented in this book for a healthful, low-fat diet, most people can dramatically reduce their blood cholesterol. Everyone over age twenty should have their cholesterol tested at least once every five years—more often, if necessary. This inset explains what blood cholesterol is, and shows you how to interpret your cholesterol test results.

Cholesterol circulates in the bloodstream in particles called *lipoproteins*. Two kinds of lipoproteins should be measured when you get your blood cholesterol tested. *Low-density lipoproteins* (LDLs) are also known as *"lethal"* or "bad" cholesterol. These cholesterol-rich particles transport cholesterol throughout the bloodstream to the cells of the body, where it is needed for various uses. If the LDLs are loaded down with more cholesterol than the cells can use, the excess can collect on artery walls, forming plaques. Plaques can eventually block arteries and cause a heart attack or stroke. *High-density lipoproteins* (HDLs) are also known as *"healthy"* or "good" cholesterol. These particles carry cholesterol away from the cells and back to the liver for recycling or disposal.

As you might guess, the worst case scenario would be to have high LDL cholesterol and low HDL cholesterol. In such a situation, unhealthfully large amounts of cholesterol would be shipped out into the bloodstream, and only very small amounts would be shipped back to the liver for disposal. This would make plenty of cholesterol available for forming plaques in the blood vessels.

Which levels of HDLs and LDLs are considered healthy, and which are considered unhealthy? The table on page 13 categorizes cholesterol, LDL, and HDL levels according to risk for heart disease.

---

one killer of Americans—is well established. And excess fat plays a central role. The most common form of cardiovascular disease is atherosclerosis, a condition in which cholesterol-rich plaques form on artery walls. As discussed earlier in this chapter, a diet high in saturated fat, trans fat, and cholesterol encourages the development of these plaques. As plaques get larger and larger over the years, they can cut off blood flow to the heart or brain, causing a heart attack or stroke. Plaques also cause artery walls to become hard and inelastic, which raises blood pressure. To make matters worse, plaque-lined arteries increase the tendency of blood to form dangerous clots as it passes through.

Unfortunately, the well-intentioned person who switches to a diet high in polyunsaturated fats may add to his or her problem. How? Certain polyunsaturated fats—such as corn, safflower, and sunflower oils, and products made from these oils—are rich in omega-6 fatty acids, which alter body chemistry to favor the development of blood clots and high blood pressure. As for monounsaturated fats, while they have no

Cholesterol, Lipoproteins, and Heart Disease Risk in Adults

Fraction Measured	Low Risk	Intermediate Risk	High Risk
Total Cholesterol	Less than 200	200–239	240 and above
LDL Cholesterol	Less than 130	130–159	160 and above
HDL Cholesterol	60 and above	35–59	Less than 35

Since your balance of LDLs and HDLs determines how much cholesterol is available to be deposited in blood vessels, your cholesterol test results will probably also list the LDL/HDL ratio or the cholesterol/HDL ratio. For the lowest risk, you should have:

☐ An LDL/HDL ratio of 3 or less, which means that you have no more than 3 times as much bad cholesterol as good cholesterol.

☐ A cholesterol/HDL ratio of 4.5 or less, which means that you have no more than 4.5 times as much total cholesterol as good cholesterol.

High blood cholesterol is just one of a number of risk factors for heart disease. Other risk factors include smoking, high blood pressure, diabetes, family history, obesity, and a sedentary lifestyle. Healthful dietary changes can dramatically reduce both blood cholesterol and your risk for heart disease, primarily by lowering LDL cholesterol. You can raise your HDL cholesterol mainly by exercising, by maintaining a healthy body weight, and by not smoking.

known harmful effects on the cardiovascular system, when too much is consumed, they can contribute to weight gain, and thus place a greater strain on the heart and blood vessels.

Just as high-fat foods should be avoided in a heart-healthy diet, certain other foods should be included in generous amounts. Dietary fiber, especially soluble fiber—found in oats, oat bran, dried beans and peas, and many vegetables and fruits—should be an important part of any eating plan. Soluble fiber helps reduce blood cholesterol levels by binding with bile acids, the raw material from which cholesterol is made. As bile acids are swept from the body along with the fiber, there is less material for making cholesterol, so that blood cholesterol concentrations drop.

Consuming a nutrient-rich diet is another strategy for bolstering your defenses against heart disease. Antioxidants like vitamin E, vitamin C, and the carotenoids are needed to deactivate the destructive free radicals that promote heart disease. Nutrients like folate, copper, and chromium are also essential for maintaining a healthy cardiovascular system. And getting plenty of calcium, potassium, and magnesium—while avoiding too much sodium—is essential for maintaining normal blood pressure. Sadly, many people's diets fall short on the nutrients they need for optimal health. Why? They consume too few vegetables and fruits, and eat too many processed foods from which the nutrients have been lost. Within these pages, you will discover how to choose foods that are not just low in fat, but also packed with heart-healthy nutrients.

Diet and Cancer

What you eat has a profound effect on your chances of developing cancer. In fact, up to 70 percent of all cancers are thought to be diet-related. Researchers believe that high-fat diets promote cancer in a number of ways. First, high-fat diets often lead to obesity, which is associated with colon, breast, and other cancers. Second, people who eat high-fat diets tend to eat more meat, high intakes of which are associated with colon and other cancers. Third, and perhaps most important, people who eat high-fat diets often eat too few vegetables, fruits, and other plant foods. These foods are loaded with antioxidants, vitamins, minerals, and phytochemicals that actively fight cancer. They also contain fiber, which speeds the passage of food through the intestines and sweeps carcinogens from the body.

The type of fat eaten also influences cancer risk. For instance, when consumed in large amounts, both saturated fats and omega-6 polyunsaturated fats like safflower oil, sunflower oil, and corn oil are especially potent cancer promoters. Conversely, the polyunsaturated omega-3 fat found in fish offers protection against cancer. Monounsaturated fats like olive oil do not appear to promote cancer.

In general, people who eat low-fat, low-meat diets with lots of fruits, vegetables, and whole grains have the lowest risk of cancer. Does this kind of diet sound familiar? It should. It is the same way of eating that protects against heart disease and other chronic and degenerative diseases.

Diet and Diabetes

Diet is a major factor in the development of diabetes for most of the 16 million people who have this disease, and diet is the cornerstone of successful treatment. The most obvious dietary component that people think of when diabetes comes to mind is sugar, as diabetes causes blood sugar concentrations to become abnormally high. Surprisingly, though, excess fat is usually an even bigger problem. Why? High-fat diets are a primary cause of obesity. And since obesity is a strong risk factor for the development of Type II (adult onset) diabetes, controlling fat is especially important for people with this disease. Moreover, for the person who already has diabetes, a high-fat diet poses a threat to much more than weight. You see, diabetes affects the way the body metabolizes fat, causing fat and cholesterol to build up in the blood more than they would in a nondiabetic person. This explains why diabetes is considered a risk factor for heart disease. As for sugar, research has demonstrated that most people with diabetes can include some sugar in their diets. (Just how much and when should be determined with the help of your nutritionist or dietitian.)

One of the most prudent dietary strategies for the control of diabetes is the adoption of a fiber-rich diet. High-fiber whole foods like whole grains, legumes, vegetables, and fruits contain nutrients such as chromium, magnesium, zinc, and B vitamins. These nutrients, which are processed out of white flour and other refined foods, help the body metabolize carbohydrates. Fibrous foods also require more chewing and are more filling and satisfying than refined foods—a real boon to people who are trying to lose weight. As a bonus, soluble fibers—found in oats, oat bran, legumes, and some other foods—help stabilize blood sugar levels.

Contrary to popular belief, a diabetic diet is not different from any other healthful diet. People with diabetes do have to be especially careful to eat the right number of calories to maintain their desired body weight, as overeating in general will promote weight gain and elevate blood sugar levels. And they have to be careful to eat consistent amounts of carbohydrates at each meal, especially if they are taking diabetes pills or insulin shots. But the best foods for people with diabetes are those that should be featured in every good diet—foods that are low in fat and sugar, high in fiber, and rich in nutrients.

This chapter has offered many important facts about fats and how they affect your health. If you're now feeling overwhelmed by information about saturated fats, omega-3 versus omega-6 fatty acids, HDLs, and LDLs, don't worry. The next chapter will make your transition to a low-fat diet a breeze. First, you will learn how to set up your own personal fat budget. Then, you will learn some simple guidelines that will help you trim the unwanted fat from your diet and add the essential nutrients that you need for the best possible health.

2. The Basics of Living Fat-Free

Chapter 1 gave you plenty of good reasons to get the fat out of your life. This chapter will help you get started on the road to success. First, you will discover how to develop your own personal fat budget. Then, with the help of some simple guidelines for good eating—as well as some easy-to-follow steps for weight loss—you will learn how to prune unwanted fat from your diet and choose the nutrient-rich foods that will promote the best possible health. In the chapters that follow, you will learn how to apply this information to every situation imaginable, from grocery shopping and cooking, to dining out, traveling, and more.

BUDGETING YOUR FAT

For most Americans, about 34 percent of the calories in their diet come from fat. However, currently it is recommended that fat calories constitute no more than 30 percent of the diet, and, in fact, 20 to 25 percent would be even better in most cases. So the amount of fat you should eat every day is based on the number of calories you need. Because people's calorie needs depend on their weight, age, gender, activity level, and metabolic rate, these needs vary greatly from person to person. Most adults, though, must consume 13 to 15 calories per pound each day to maintain their weight. Of course, some people need even fewer calories, while very physically active people need more.

Once you have determined your calorie requirements, you can estimate a fat budget for yourself. Suppose you are a moderately active person who weighs 150 pounds. You will probably need about 15 calories per pound to maintain your weight, or about 2,250 calories per day. To limit your fat intake to 20 percent of your calorie intake, you can eat no more than 450 calories derived from fat per day (2,250 x .20 = 450). To convert this to grams of fat, divide by 9, as one gram of fat has 9 calories. Therefore, you should limit yourself to 50 grams of fat per day (450 ÷ by 9 = 50).

The following table shows two maximum daily fat-gram budgets—one based on 20 percent of calorie intake, and one based on 25 percent of calorie intake. If you are overweight, go by the weight you would like to be. This will allow you to gradually reach your goal weight. And keep in mind that although you have budgeted X amount of fat grams per day, you don't have to eat that amount of fat—you just have to avoid going over budget.

Recommended Daily Calorie and Fat Intakes

Weight (pounds)	Recommended Daily Calorie Intake (13-15 cals per lb.)	Daily Fat-Gram Intake (20% of Caloric Intake)	Daily Fat-Gram Intake (25% of Caloric Intake)
100	1,300–1500	29–33	36–42
110	1,430–1,650	32–37	40–46
120	1,560–1,800	34–40	43–50
130	1,690–1,950	38–43	47–54
140	1,820–2,100	40–46	51–58
150	1,950–2,250	43–50	54–62
160	2,080–2,400	46–53	58–67
170	2,210–2,550	49–57	61–71
180	2,340–2,700	52–60	65–75
190	2,470–2,850	55–63	69–79
200	2,600–3,000	58–66	72–83

REMEMBER THAT CALORIES COUNT, TOO

Weight loss is the number-one reason that most people try to reduce their fat intake. And since low-fat foods are generally also low in calories, a low-fat diet *can* help you reach and maintain a healthy body weight—unless you eat too many fat-free sweets and junk foods.

Many people mistakenly think that if a food is low in fat or fat-free, they can consume unlimited quantities of it. They may start their day with a fat-free muffin, keep a jar of jelly beans or hard candy on their desk to nibble on throughout the day, snack on low-fat cookies at break time, and eat a bowl of fat-free ice cream topped with fat-free chocolate syrup for an evening snack. Although all of these foods are better choices than their full-fat counterparts, they are loaded with sugar and provide few or no nutrients. Moreover, some of these items have just as many calories as their full-fat counterparts.

The truth is that *any* foods eaten in excess of calories burned in a day will be converted to body fat. So if you are trying to lose weight, stay within the bounds of your fat budget and choose mostly nutrient-rich foods. By doing this, you should be able to reach your weight-management goals. But if you have trouble losing or maintaining your weight, consider whether you are staying within the bounds of your calorie budget, as well. (For more weight-loss strategies, see the inset "Simple Steps to Successful Weight Loss" on page 19.)

Simple Steps to Successful Weight Loss

When most people begin a weight-loss diet, they do so with monumental effort—and then quickly run out of steam. In their zeal to get off to a quick start, many dieters eat such ridiculously small amounts of food that they feel weak, hungry, and deprived. Many also spend long hours in the kitchen chopping, measuring, and cooking special diet foods, only to find that after a few weeks, the diet is just too much work to continue. Whatever the reason for their failure, 95 percent of all dieters abandon their diets before reaching their goal weight and soon regain the lost weight—plus a few additional pounds.

What's a dieter to do? Relax. Forget about special weight-loss diets, stop being a slave to the scale, and, above all, be patient. Concentrate on developing healthier habits, and weight loss will follow. Weight that is lost gradually, as the result of modest lifestyle changes, is much more likely to stay off than is weight lost on a quick-fix diet. Here are some simple tips that will help you get started on the road to successful weight loss.

☐ Choose low-fat, fiber-rich foods. Watching your fat grams will help keep calories under control. Eating plenty of fiber—in vegetables, fruits, whole grains, and legumes—will help you feel full and satisfied. In fact, serving large portions of vegetables and fruits at each meal is one of the secrets of successful weight loss. The reason? Besides being high in fiber and supernutritious, vegetables are very low in calories. People who skip the vegetables and fruits at a mere 25 to 50 calories per cup, and pile on extra rice or pasta at 200 calories per cup, may find weight loss slower than they expected. (Realize that starchy vegetables like corn, peas, lima beans, and potatoes contain about the same amount of calories as pasta and rice, so be careful not to overdo portions of these veggies.)

☐ Eat balanced meals. One of the biggest mistakes that people make when adopting a low-fat diet is to entirely cut out protein-rich foods, such as fish, poultry, lean meats, legumes, soy products, and dairy products. Instead, they go overboard on pasta, bread, and other starches. While it's important not to eat too much protein, including some *low-fat* protein in each meal will help you feel fuller longer, and will provide the essential amino acids needed to maintain and repair the body. An easy way to be sure you are getting a balanced meal is to mentally divide your plate into fourths. Then fill a quarter of your plate with a protein-rich food; fill another quarter with a starchy food; and fill the remaining half with vegetables and fruits.

☐ Limit sugar. Sugary foods—even fat-free versions—are loaded with calories. Sugary foods also contain few or no nutrients, and when eaten in excess, they can deplete your body of essential nutrients like chromium and the B vitamins. Read labels for sugar content, keeping in mind that every four grams of sugar is equal to one teaspoon.

☐ Eat at least three meals per day, spacing them out evenly. Eating just one or two meals a day slows your metabolism, and increases the likelihood that your meals will be stored as body fat. Eating several meals throughout the day will help keep your metabolism going strong.

☐ Do not overwhelm yourself with cooking, weighing, and measuring foods. Try one or two new low-fat recipes a week. When you find a recipe that works for you, make it a regular part of your diet. Continue experimenting with new recipes and new foods at your own pace, phasing in the new and phasing out the old. Before you know it, you will have designed your own personal low-fat diet.

☐ Eat when you are hungry, but learn the difference between hunger and other physical sensations. People often overeat because they confuse hunger with thirst, fatigue, or stress. If you keep properly hydrated with six to eight glasses of water each day, get enough rest, and work to keep stress under control, you will be less likely to overeat.

☐ Eat slowly. As you eat, hormones and other chemicals are generated by your digestive system. These chemicals eventually make their way to the brain, which then lets you know that you have had enough to eat. Since it takes about twenty minutes for this to happen, people who eat quickly consume more food and more calories than they need before they begin to feel full.

☐ Don't forget to exercise. The two main predictors for weight-loss success are low-fat eating and exercise. By both decreasing your dietary fat and calories and regularly exercising, you will maximize your chance for long-term success. Exercise doesn't merely burn extra calories. It also helps you gain muscle and lose fat, which, in turn, raises your metabolism and improves your ability to burn calories all day long. As a bonus, exercise helps reduce stress—a major cause of overeating.

Small changes like the ones described above can make a big fat difference in your weight. For instance, by eliminating just 100 calories from your diet on a daily basis—the equivalent of one tablespoon of butter, mayonnaise, or other fat—you can lose ten pounds in a year. By eating a turkey sandwich for lunch instead of a deluxe cheese burger, you can lose twenty pounds in a year. Substitute water for those two daily high-sugar sodas, and lose thirty pounds. Or walk five miles a week, and lose seven pounds. Changes like these, maintained for long periods of time, take weight off permanently. Need more help with your weight loss program? A registered dietitian, nutritionist, or other qualified health professional can help you determine a healthy goal weight, and guide you in modifying your diet and lifestyle in a way that will allow you to reach your goal.

THE GUIDELINES FOR GOOD EATING

Once you have arrived at daily calorie and fat budgets, you can begin pruning unwanted fat from your diet. This task is easier than it sounds once you become acquainted with a few guidelines for good eating. The following are some simple but very effective strategies that will help you not only manage your weight, but also maximize your nutrients and promote optimum health.

Choose Lean Meats, Poultry, and Seafood, and Limit Portions to Six Ounces or Less Per Day

Meats contribute more fat and cholesterol to the average diet than does any other food group. Does this mean that you are doomed to a diet of dried-out skinless chicken breasts? Absolutely not! In Chapter 4, you will discover how to select red meats, poultry, and even lunchmeats that have just a fraction of the fat found in their full-fat counterparts. You may question why it's necessary to limit portion size to six ounces when so many lean meats are available. The fact is that even lean meats contain cholesterol. By keeping portions modest in size, you will insure that your cholesterol intake remains below the recommended limit of 300 milligrams per day. This guideline will also help you leave room on your plate for the nutrient- and fiber-rich vegetables, grains, and fruits that should make up the biggest part of your diet.

Where do fish and seafood fit in? These foods range from practically fat-free to moderately fatty. However, the oil in fish provides an essential kind of fat—known as omega-3 fatty acids—that most people's diets do not provide in sufficient amounts. (See pages 5 to 8 for more information about essential fatty acids.) Therefore, all kinds of fish—even the more oily ones like salmon and mackerel—are considered healthful, and are excellent alternatives to meat and poultry. In fact, fish should be substituted for meat several times a week.

The emphasis on limiting meat to six ounces or less per day may lead you to think that it would be best to totally eliminate this food group. The fact is that you can eliminate meat, poultry, and seafood from your diet if you prefer. However, when you eliminate these foods, you must substitute a protein-rich alternative like legumes, which are discussed below, or a soy product such as tofu. These foods provide protein as well as many of the same minerals that meat does, insuring nutritional balance.

Substitute Legumes for Meat Often

The best way to keep meat portions modest in size is to substitute legumes—dried beans and peas—for meat as often as possible. Legumes are rich in protein and potassium, and provide many of the same nutrients found in meats. In addition, these tasty morsels contain little or no fat, are cholesterol-free, and are loaded with cholesterol-lowering soluble fiber. Moreover, beans help stabilize blood sugar levels and provide a feeling of fullness that helps prevent overeating. If this isn't reason enough to eat more legumes, consider that beans and peas are among the most economical foods you can buy. So substituting legumes for meat can have a big impact not only on your health, but also on your grocery bill.

One type of legume that is gaining popularity in this country is the soybean. Once relegated only to health foods stores, a wide variety of soy products can now be found at your grocery store. Tofu, tofu crumbles, texturized vegetable protein, and even burgers and crumbled ground meat alternatives made with soy protein are all widely available. Chapter 4 provides more information on selecting these healthful meat alternatives. And if you don't know how to use legumes in your meals, turn to Chapter 6, which offers plenty of ways to make legumes a delicious part of your low-fat diet.

Choose Nonfat and Low-Fat Dairy Products

Like meats, dairy products have long been a major source of fat and cholesterol in the average diet. Fortunately, this no longer has to be true. Chapter 4 will introduce you to a delightful variety of nonfat and low-fat products that can beautifully replace full-fat cheeses, sour cream, and other popular foods. These new products not only will eliminate excess calories and artery-clogging saturated fat from your diet, but, by providing nutrients such as calcium and potassium, will help guard against osteoporosis, high blood pressure, and many other health problems.

Limit Your Use of Table and Cooking Fats

Fats used for cooking and baking—like butter and margarine—and fats added at the table—oily salad dressings, mayonnaise, and butter, for instance—can really add up. In fact, in their full-fat versions, just one tablespoon of any of these products will add about 10 grams of fat to your meal. The good news is that for each of these foods, there is now a no- or low-fat alternative that can help you greatly reduce or eliminate the fats you use in cooking, in baking, and at the table. Chapter 4 will introduce you to many of these exciting new products, and Chapters 5 and 6 will show you how to use them to create great-tasting dishes that your whole family will love.

Limit Your Sodium Intake to 2,400 Milligrams Per Day

A limited sodium intake has many benefits, ranging from better-controlled blood pressure to stronger bones. But of all the guidelines for good eating, this one can be the most difficult to follow, since many low-fat and fat-free foods contain extra salt.

Fortunately, with a just a little effort, even this dietary goal can be met. The most effective sodium-control strategy is to avoid using salt for cooking and at the table. Believe it or not, just one teaspoon of salt contains 2,300 milligrams of sodium—almost your entire daily allowance—so it pays to put the salt shaker away. Another effective strategy is to limit your intake of high-sodium processed foods. Read labels, and choose the lower-sodium frozen meals, canned goods, broths, cheeses, and other products. Also, whenever you make a recipe that contains high-sodium cheeses, processed meats, or other salty ingredients, be sure not to add any extra salt. The recipes in this book will show you how to balance high-sodium products with low-sodium ingredients, herbs, and spices to make dishes that are low in sodium but high in flavor.

Choose Whole Grains Over Refined Grains

Largely because of the widespread use of refined grains—white-flour products and white rice, for instance—the average diet falls short of the 25 or more grams of dietary fiber recommended for daily consumption. Yet when changing your diet to promote good health, the importance of low-fat foods is rivaled only by the importance of fiber. Dietary fiber helps control blood cholesterol and blood sugar, and helps protect against colon cancer. Watching your weight? While a diet of refined, low-fiber foods will leave you feeling hungry, a high-fiber eating plan will keep you feeling full and satisfied. This is one of the reasons that several major weight-loss programs now emphasize the importance of low-fat, high-fiber eating.

But low fiber is just one of the problems posed by refined grains. The refining process strips grains of most of their nutrients. Whole grains, on the other hand, provide folate, vitamins B_6 and E, chromium, magnesium, and a host of other disease-protective nutrients.

People who are not used to eating high-fiber foods should add these foods to their diets gradually. Why? Some people may experience bloating and gas when they begin a high-fiber regimen—although this usually diminishes in a few weeks as the body becomes accustomed to eating whole, natural foods. When following a high-fiber diet, it is also important to drink at least six to eight cups of water per day. Fiber needs to absorb water in order to move smoothly through the digestive system and exert its beneficial effects.

When made properly, breads, muffins, casseroles, breakfast foods, side dishes, soups, and even desserts can include wholesome whole grains. Chapter 4 recommends a variety of versatile, fiber-rich grain products that can be found in your grocery store, while Chapter 6 offers tempting recipes that show you how to use these and other foods to create hearty and wholesome dishes in your own kitchen.

Eat At Least Five Servings of Fruits and Vegetables Every Day

Fruits and vegetables offer a bounty of nutrients, fiber, and substances known as phytochemicals—all powerful preventive medicines against cancer, heart disease, and many other health problems. Since not all of the protective substances present in these foods have been identified, and some of them probably never will be, it is impossible to get all the benefits of fruits and vegetables from vitamin pills. So fruits and vegetables can and should be served in generous amounts at every meal.

Sadly, studies show that the average American eats only about three servings of vegetables and fruits each day. Even worse, much of the time, these foods are laden with butter, margarine, cheese sauce, or other fats. But, as the remaining chapters in this book will show, getting your five-a-day is not as hard as you may think—even when eating away from home. Also, you may not realize that a serving is really quite small. A medium-sized piece of fruit, a half cup of cooked or raw fruit or vegetables, a cup of leafy salad greens, a quarter cup of dried fruit, or three fourths of a cup of fruit juice each constitute a serving. So if you include at least one cup of fruit or vegetables at each meal, you will be well on your way to five-a-day.

Finally, remember that five servings are the *minimum* recommended amount. To maximize your health, aim for seven to nine servings.

Eat Sugar Only in Moderation

When people start reducing their fat intake, often, without really thinking about it, they greatly increase their sugar intake. This is easy to understand. Stroll down the aisles of your local grocery store, and you will see a mind-boggling array of fat-free cookies, brownies, ice creams, and other goodies. While these products may contain little or no fat, they usually contain as much sugar as their high-fat counterparts—and sometimes more!

What health threats are posed by sugar? First and foremost, sugar contains no nutrients, and, when eaten in excess, can actually deplete your body's stores of chromium, the B vitamins, and other vitamins and minerals. Second, people often eat sugary foods instead of nutritious foods—a practice that contributes to nutritional deficiencies. Third, by overwhelming the taste buds and increasing our threshold for sweet flavors, diets rich in sugary foods can cause us to lose our taste for the more subtle flavors of wholesome, natural foods. Finally, sugary foods are usually loaded with calories, making them a real menace if you're watching your weight.

The good news is that, in moderation, sugar can be enjoyed without harm to your health. What's a moderate amount? No more than 10 percent of your daily intake of calories should come from sugar. For a person who needs 2,000 calories a day to maintain his or her weight, this amounts to an upper limit of 50 grams, or 12.5 teaspoons (about a quarter cup), of sugar a day. If you need only 1,600 calories a day, your upper limit would be 40 grams, or 10 teaspoons. Naturally, a diet that is lower in sugar is even better. To put your sugar budget into perspective, the following table lists the sugar content of selected foods in both grams and teaspoons.

Sugar Content of Selected Foods

Food	Amount	Sugar (grams)	Sugar (teaspoons)
Apple pie	1/8 pie	24	6
Chocolate bar	1 1/2 ounces	24	6
Chocolate cake with icing	1/16 cake	34	8 1/2
Fat-free brownie	1 brownie	18	4 1/2
Fat-free cereal bar	1 bar	17	4 1/4
Fruit toaster pastry	1 pastry	16	4
Jellybeans	1/2 cup	79	20
Low-fat cream-filled sandwich cookies	2 cookies	12	3
Nonfat ice cream	1 cup	32	8
Soft drink	12 ounces	38	9 1/2

While the guidelines for good eating are few in number, they can make a big difference both in your diet and in the way you look and feel. And you'll find that the tips provided throughout this book make it surprisingly easy to follow these guidelines and build a healthful, enjoyable diet.

3. Reading a Food Label

Stroll down the aisle of any supermarket, and you're likely to see a common phenomenon: people staring with rapt attention at cans, boxes, and jars. The reason? They're trying to decipher the Nutrition Facts food labels.

Almost all food products today must, by law, provide certain nutrition facts on their labels. The only foods that do not have to list this information are foods sold in bulk; foods produced by small businesses; foods created to meet the needs of certain medical conditions; spices and other foods that contain insignificant amounts of nutrients; and fresh meats, seafood, and poultry.

While the Nutrition Facts food labels were designed to give you the information you need to make wise food choices, in truth, many people are still baffled by much of the data presented on these labels. If you count yourself among this group, this chapter is for you. In the following pages, you will learn to interpret each component of the Nutrition Facts label, and you will see how this component fits into a healthy diet. You will discover that the Nutrition Facts label can be an invaluable guide that allows you to zero in on the best products available—products that can help you meet your personal weight and nutrition goals. In fact, you'll find that reading and understanding a food label is another great secret of fat-free living.

COMPONENTS OF THE NUTRITION FACTS LABEL

Each component of the Nutrition Facts label contains important information that can help you meet your nutrition goals. However, unless you understand some nutrition "basics," this information can seem overwhelming and confusing. This section will share the secrets of deciphering even the most confusing of labels, enabling you to quickly glean the most significant facts and apply them to your own personal needs.

Serving Size

It is crucial to understand what the manufacturer calls a serving, and to see how this compares with what you call a serving. This information should, of course, be kept in mind when evaluating the remaining nutrition data. Why? Although a fat or sodium count may seem fine when, for instance, only a quarter of the package is considered,

Nutrition Facts

Serving Size ½ cup (114g)
Servings Per Container 4

Amount Per Serving

Calories 90   Calories from Fat 30

	% Daily Value*
Total Fat 3g	5%
Saturated fat 0g	0%
Cholesterol 0mg	0%
Sodium 300mg	13%
Total Carbohydrate 13g	4%
Dietary Fiber 3g	12%
Sugars 3g	
Protein 3g	

Vitamin A 80% • Vitamin C 60% • Calcium 4% • Iron 4%

*Percent Daily Values are based on
a 2,000 calorie diet. Your Daily
Values may be higher or lower
depending on your calorie needs:

Nutrient		2,000 Calories	2,500 Calories
Total fat	Less than	65g	80g
Sat Fat	Less than	20g	25g
Cholesterol	Less than	300mg	300mg
Sodium	Less than	2,400mg	2,400mg
Total Carbohydrate		300g	375g
Fiber		25g	30g

Calories per gram:
Fat 9 • Carbohydrates 4 • Protein 4

Sodium. Limit yourself to 2,400 milligrams per day.

Protein. Aim for .36 gram per pound of ideal body weight per day.

Nutrients. Expressed as a percentage of the Daily Value—a recommended daily amount based on a 2,000-calorie diet—this may not reflect your personal requirements.

Calories. Compare the calories per serving to your personal calorie budget to see how the food fits into your diet.

Calories From Fat. This figure tells you how many of the calories in the product are contributed by fat. Your diet should get no more than 20% to 25% of its calories from fat. If you stick to your fat budget, this will automatically fall into place.

Dietary Fiber. Aim for at least 25 grams per day.

Sugar. Limit yourself to 50 grams of refined sugar per day. Realize that this number doesn't discriminate between natural, higher-nutrient fruit and milk sugars, and nutrient-poor refined sugars.

Daily Values Percentages and Footnotes. Both the Daily Value footnotes provided at the bottom of the label and the % Daily Value data found higher on the label assume a diet of either 2,000 or 2,500 calories. Also, the Daily Value for fat assumes you want to limit fat to 30% of calorie intake. If you're aiming for fewer calories or less fat, this information will overestimate your needs.

Serving Size. Similar foods (like cereals, cookies, etc.) have similar serving sizes. Be sure to compare the manufacturer's serving size with what you call a serving.

Total Fat. Compare the fat grams per serving to your personal fat budget to see how the food fits into your diet.

Saturated Fat. This should constitute no more than ⅓ of your total fat budget. Realize that artery-clogging trans fats are not included in this number, but are part of the total figure.

Cholesterol. Limit yourself to 300 milligrams per day.

The Nutrition Facts Label at a Glance

if your idea of a portion is half of the package, the fat and sodium values may prove to be unhealthfully high.

Calories Per Serving

If you have not already done so, use the table on page 18 to determine your daily calorie budget. Then, keeping the manufacturer's definition of a serving in mind, see how the product fits into your calorie budget.

Total Fat Per Serving

To understand this information, you first must determine your daily fat-gram budget. (Again, see the table on page 18.) Then, again keeping in mind the manufacturer's serving size, evaluate how this food fits into your fat budget.

Percentage of Daily Value

In the case of certain dietary components—total fat, for instance—the amount is expressed not only in grams or milligrams, but also as a percentage of the Daily Value, a recommended daily amount based on a diet of 2,000 calories. When reading these Daily Value figures, keep in mind that if your calorie budget is more or less than 2,000 calories a day, these percentages will not hold true for you. Just as important, remember that the Daily Value for fat assumes that your fat budget is 30 percent of your total calories. If you prefer a more prudent 20- or 25-percent fat budget, the Daily Value figure may lead you to overestimate your fat allowance.

Calories From Fat

Besides listing the calories and total fat grams in one serving of a product, the Nutrition Facts label tells you how many of the calories in a serving of the product come from fat. This figure is derived by multiplying the total fat grams by 9. (Each gram of fat provides 9 calories.)

While some people use the calories-from-fat information to calculate the percentage of calories that come from fat, remember that it is not necessary for every food in your diet to derive only 20 or 25 percent of its total calories from fat. If you stick to your fat budget and just count total fat grams, your diet will balance out. This means that even a food like peanut butter—which gets a whopping 76 percent of its calories from fat!—has a place in a healthy diet as long as you compensate by eating lower-fat foods throughout the day.

Saturated Fat

Besides listing the total fat grams per serving, the Nutrition Facts label tells you how much of the total fat is saturated fat. This is worth looking at because saturated fat is the kind that raises blood cholesterol levels and promotes heart disease. Saturated fat should constitute no more than one third of your total fat intake. So if your fat budget allows, say, 45 grams of fat per day, no more than 15 grams of this fat should be saturated. Of course, less saturated fat would be even better.

Bear in mind that trans fats, which are found in margarines and other solid shortening, raise cholesterol levels just as much as saturated fats do. These fats, however, are not listed separately on the food label. Instead, they are included in the figure for total fat. This means that if a food contains partially hydrogenated vegetable oil, the label underestimates the cholesterol-raising potential of the food.

Cholesterol

The recommended daily limit for this substance, which is found only in animal products, is 300 milligrams per day. By choosing nonfat and low-fat dairy products, limiting your meat portions to 6 ounces or less per day, limiting egg yolks to 4 per week, and keeping your eye out for high cholesterol counts, you should be able to stay well within your budget.

Sodium

The recommended daily limit for sodium is 2,400 milligrams per day. Since so many processed foods are high in salt, it makes sense to check food labels for sodium counts and to avoid any foods with excessively high values.

Dietary Fiber

Fiber, a type of carbohydrate found only in grains, fruits, and vegetables, is listed under the "Total Carbohydrate" section of the Nutrition Facts label. Aim for at least 25 grams of fiber per day, and choose your products accordingly.

Sugars

Like fiber, sugars are found under "Total Carbohydrate." Because no more than 10 percent of your calories should come from refined sugar, you should probably limit yourself to no more than 40 to 50 grams per day. Keep in mind, though, that the Nutrition Facts figure given for sugar includes both refined sweeteners and the sugar that occurs naturally in fruits and milk. Because the sugar in fruit and milk comes packaged with nutrients and fiber, it should not be lumped in with refined sweeteners. Remember this when evaluating products like breakfast cereals and yogurt, which may derive some or much of their sugar from fruit and other wholesome ingredients.

Protein

Unlike most of the other nutrients, protein is not expressed as a percentage of the Daily Value. How do you know if you are getting enough of this nutrient? Most people need about 0.36 gram of protein per pound of ideal body weight. So if your ideal weight is 150 pounds, you will need about of 54 grams of protein per day ($150 \times .36 = 54$). While it is important to eat your complete allotment of protein, many Americans eat twice as much protein as they need, and protein excesses can contribute to kidney disease, osteoporosis, and other disorders. By following the strategies outlined in the guidelines for good eating, you will get all the protein your body needs for good health, but not more than your body can handle.

Nutrients

The Nutrition Facts label provides information on the vitamin A, vitamin C, calcium, and iron contents of a food. These values are expressed as a percentage of Daily

Values, the recommended daily amount based on a 2,000-calorie diet. As the label warns, your needs may be higher or lower for certain nutrients.

Ingredients

This portion of the label—which is not a part of the Nutrition Facts section—lists a product's ingredients in order of quantity (by weight). Those ingredients listed first are present in the greatest amount. So if sugar, white flour, or fat is the number-one ingredient, you'll know that the food does not merit a prominent place in your diet.

WHAT YOU SEE IS WHAT YOU GET—MOST OF THE TIME

Besides the basic components of the Nutrition Facts label, food labels often use certain terms to describe a product. In the past, these terms were used inconsistently and often misleadingly. However, with the new food labels, they must now must be applied uniformly to insure that they mean the same thing on all products. Following are definitions of the most commonly used terms, as well as some cautions that will help you steer clear of common pitfalls.

Free. The product contains virtually none of a particular nutrient. (Beware, though: Just because a food is fat-free does not mean it is calorie-free, sugar-free, or sodium-free. Always read the entire label to see how other nutrients stack up.) The following specific terms are used:

Calorie Free. The product has less than 5 calories per serving.

Cholesterol Free. The product has less than 2 milligrams of cholesterol and no more than 2 grams of saturated fat per serving.

Fat Free. The product has less than 0.5 gram of fat per serving. (Beware: Fat-free does not necessarily mean low-calorie.)

Sodium Free. The product has less than 5 milligrams of sodium per serving.

Sugar Free. The product has less than 0.5 gram of sugar per serving. (Beware: Many sugar-free foods contain extra fat.)

Low. The product is low enough in a particular nutrient to allow frequent use with little danger of exceeding the recommended Daily Value. (Again, read the entire label whenever foods are labeled "low." Just because a food is low in sodium, for instance, does not mean it is low in calories, sugar, or fat.) Here are the specific terms you'll find on food labels:

Low Calorie. The product has no more than 40 calories per serving.

Low Fat. The product has no more than 3 grams of fat per serving. (Beware: Low-fat does not necessarily mean low-calorie.) There are exceptions to this rule. Frozen entrées, for instance, are allowed to have 3 grams of fat for every 3.5

ounces. So if an entrée weighs 10 ounces, it can contain up to 8.5 grams of fat and still be called low-fat.

Low Saturated Fat. The product has no more than 1 gram of saturated fat per serving, and no more than 15 percent of calories from saturated fat. In addition, no more than 1 percent of its total fat can be a trans fat. The exceptions to this rule include frozen entrées and meals, which can contain up to 1 gram of saturated fat for every 3.5 ounces.

Low Cholesterol. The product has no more than 20 milligrams of cholesterol and 2 grams of saturated fat per serving.

Low Sodium. The product has no more than 140 milligrams of sodium per serving.

Light (or Lite). This term could mean several different things. The light product could have a third less calories than the higher-calorie version, or it could contain no more than half the fat of the higher-fat version. (The label will specify which is true.)

"Light" can also refer to a product that has, at most, half the sodium of its higher-sodium counterpart. If this is the case, the product must say "light in sodium." However, if the light-in-sodium food is also a low-fat or low-calorie food, it can just be called "light."

The word "light" can also appear on products like brown sugar, corn syrup, and molasses to describe the product's color.

Reduced or Less. The product has at least 25 percent less of a nutrient such as fat, sodium, sugar, or calories than does the original version of the product.

Percent Fat Free. This term, which can be used only on foods that are low-fat or fat-free, refers to the percentage of a food by weight that is free of fat. For example, if 100 grams (about 3.5 ounces) of a particular brand of turkey bologna contain 3 grams of fat, the product can bear a label stating that it is 97 percent fat-free.

A word of warning is in order. Some people get "percent fat-free" confused with "percent of calories from fat." These are not the same thing. For instance, if a brand of 95-percent fat-free turkey bologna contains 80 calories and 2.5 grams of fat per serving, it gets 28 percent of its calories from fat—even though it is 95 percent fat-free by weight. How can this be? A good portion of the weight of bologna is made up of water. In fact, manufacturer's sometimes add water to products to reduce the percentage of fat per serving! Of course, water contains no calories, so that when looking at only the calorie-providing portion of the bologna, you find that fat provides well over 5 percent of the product's calories.

Don't get caught up comparing these two figures, or you might never get out of the grocery store. As long as you stay within your fat gram budget for the day, calories from fat and percentage of calories from fat will fall into place.

Lean. Found on packaged seafood and cooked meat and poultry products, this term indicates that the product has less than 10 grams of total fat, less than 4 grams of saturated fat, and less than 95 milligrams of cholesterol per serving.

Extra Lean. Also found on packaged seafood and cooked meat and poultry products, this indicates that the product has less than 5 grams of total fat, less than 2 grams of saturated fat, and less than 95 milligrams of cholesterol per serving.

Reduced Cholesterol. The product has at least 25 percent less cholesterol than the higher-cholesterol version, and no more than 2 grams of saturated fat per serving.

Good Source. The product provides 10 to 19 percent of the Daily Value for a particular nutrient.

High, Rich In, or Excellent Source. The product contains at least 20 percent of the Daily Value for that nutrient.

More. The product provides at least 10 percent more of a desirable nutrient than does a similar product.

Very Low Sodium. The product contains no more than 35 milligrams of sodium per serving.

Reduced Sodium. The product has at least 25 percent less sodium per serving than does the higher-sodium version.

High Fiber. The product provides at least 5 grams of fiber per serving.

Good Source of Fiber. The product provides 2.5 to 4.9 grams of fiber per serving.

THE BOTTOM LINE ON FOOD LABELS

If you feel that the Nutrition Facts label provides more information than you need—or want—to know, take heart. You don't have to memorize the definitions of countless terms or understand Daily Values to shop smart. As long as you know your own personal fat and calorie budgets, and keep in mind the budgets discussed in Chapter 2 for cholesterol (less than 300 milligrams per day), sodium (less than 2,400 milligrams per day), sugar (less than 50 grams of added refined sugar per day), and fiber (25 or more grams per day), you are ready to do some healthy grocery shopping. And the next chapter—an aisle-by-aisle guide to the supermarket—will help you do just that.

4. Supermarket Strategies for Living Fat-Free

The past few years have brought a revolution to the supermarket. Literally thousands of new low- and no-fat products have emerged in response to consumer demand. In fact, there is now a low- or no-fat alternative to just about anything you can think of. Certainly, eating healthfully has never been easier or more enjoyable. Nor has it been more overwhelming—because along with the wholesome low-fat products has come a flood of fat-free junk foods. And a diet that includes too much of the latter can contribute to excess weight as well as to poor health.

How can you tell the difference between wholesome low- and no-fat foods and fat-free junk foods? And how can you choose products that will help you get the fat out of your dishes *without* eliminating the tastes and textures you love? That is what this chapter is all about. For every department, from the meat and dairy cases, to the baked goods and the cereal and snack aisles, you will find recommendations for specific brand name products, as well as fat-fighting strategies that will help you zero in on those foods that will best meet your dietary needs. As you start using the suggested products and become familiar with their labels, you will become a whiz at picking out the best of the new foods as they enter the market. This chapter also offers plenty of tips for using low- and no-fat products in cooking and meal planning. (For more information on cutting the fat from your recipes, see Chapter 5.)

THE DAIRY CASE

The dairy case offers an amazing array of fat-free and low-fat products—each one a great way to dramatically cut back on dietary fat. This section highlights some of the available products, and provides simple guidelines for choosing and using the best of these products.

Bear in mind that unlike most areas of the food industry, the dairy business is partially constituted of local and regional manufacturers. Therefore, each part of the country has many fine brands that are specific to that region. Most grocery chains also carry their own store brands of nonfat and low-fat dairy foods. By comparing your local products with the national brands highlighted below, you will be able to choose those foods that best meet your nutritional needs, your cooking needs, your tastes, and your budget.

Firm and Hard Cheeses

Both low-fat and nonfat cheeses of many types—including Swiss, Cheddar, Monterey jack, Parmesan, provolone, and mozzarella—are widely available in grocery stores. Reduced-fat cheeses generally have 3 to 6 grams of fat and 60 to 80 calories per ounce, while nonfat cheeses contain about 40 calories per ounce, and no fat at all. Compare this with whole-milk varieties, which contain 9 to 10 grams of fat and 100 to 110 calories per ounce, and you'll realize your savings.

Firm and hard cheeses can be grouped into one of two categories—natural or process. Natural cheeses generally contain 30 to 50 percent less salt than process brands. They also contain few or no artificial ingredients. Process cheeses, on the other hand, tend to be high in both salt and artificial ingredients. Process cheeses—which are so labelled for easy identification—do melt exceptionally well, though, and so are your best bet for making recipes like cheese sauces. When shopping for fat-free cheeses, look for brands like Alpine Lace Fat-Free, Borden Fat-Free, Healthy Choice, Kraft Free, Polly-O Free, Smart Beat, and Weight Watchers Fat-Free. As for reduced-fat brands, Alpine Lace Reduced-Fat, Borden Light, Cracker Barrel $^1/_3$ Less Fat, Kraft $^1/_3$ Less Fat, Sargento Light, Velveeta Light, and Weight Watchers Reduced-Fat are all widely available. (For tips on cooking with nonfat and low-fat cheeses, see Chapter 5.)

Soft Cheeses

Low-fat and nonfat cottage cheese, cream cheese, ricotta, and farmer cheese make possible a wide range of healthy delights, from low-fat lasagna to cheesecake. By understanding the differences between the various products on the market, you'll be able to pick the one that best suits your needs. For more ideas on using these products in recipes, see Chapter 5.

Cottage Cheese. Although often thought of as a diet food, full-fat cottage cheese has 5 grams of fat per 4-ounce serving, making it far from diet fare. Instead, choose nonfat or low-fat cottage cheese. Puréed until smooth, these healthful products make a great base for dips and spreads, and add richness and body to casseroles, quiches, cheesecakes, and many other recipes. Select brands with 1 percent or less milk fat, such as Breakstone's Free and Light n' Lively Nonfat. Most brands of cottage cheese are quite high in sodium, with about 400 milligrams per half cup, so it is best to avoid adding salt whenever this cheese is a recipe ingredient. As an alternative, use unsalted cottage cheese, which is available in some stores. Another option when buying cottage cheese is dry curd cottage cheese. This nonfat version is made without the "dressing" or creaming mixture. Minus the dressing, cottage cheese has a drier consistency; hence its name, dry curd. Unlike most cottage cheese, dry curd is very low in sodium. Use dry curd cottage cheese as you would nonfat cottage cheese in casseroles, quiches, dips, spreads, salad dressings, and cheesecakes. Look for brands like Breakstone's Dry Curd.

Cream Cheese. Cream cheese has long been touted as a lower-fat alternative to butter, but at 10 grams of fat per ounce (enough for both halves of a bagel), it is far from low-fat fare. Fortunately, light alternatives abound. Choose from Neufchâtel cheese, with 6 grams of fat per ounce; light cream cheese, with 3 to 5 grams of fat per ounce; and nonfat cream cheese, with no fat at all. Like Neufchâtel and light cream cheese, nonfat cream cheese may be used in dips, spreads, and sauces. Look for brands like Philadelphia Free and Healthy Choice, and use the block-style cheese for best results when following recipes. The softer tub-style nonfat cream cheese should be reserved for spreading on bagels and other foods.

Ricotta Cheese. Ricotta is a mild, slightly sweet, creamy cheese that may be used in dips, spreads, and traditional Italian dishes like lasagna. As the name implies, nonfat ricotta contains no fat at all. Low-fat and light ricottas, on the other hand, have 1 to 3 grams of fat per ounce, while whole milk ricotta has 4 grams of fat per ounce. Look for brands like Frigo Fat-Free, Polly-O Free, Maggio Nonfat, Sorrento Fat-Free, and Sargento Light. Many stores and regional dairies offer their own fat-free brands as well.

Soft Curd Farmer Cheese. This soft, spreadable white cheese makes a good low-fat substitute for cream cheese. Brands made with skim milk have about 3 grams of fat per ounce compared with cream cheese's 10 grams. Some stores also carry nonfat brands. Soft curd farmer cheese may be used in dips, spreads, and cheesecakes, and as a filling for blintzes. Some brands are made with whole milk, so read the label before you buy. Look for a brand like Friendship Farmer Cheese.

Nondairy Cheese Alternatives

If you choose to avoid dairy products because of a lactose intolerance or for another reason, you'll be glad to know that low-fat cheeses made from soymilk, almond milk, and Brazil nut milk are now available in a variety of flavors. Look for brands like AlmondRella, VeganRella, TofuRella, Soya Kaas, Nu Tofu, and Smart Beat Fat Free Nondairy Slices. Be aware that some of these brands do contain casein, a milk protein that you may want to avoid.

Other Low-Fat and Nonfat Dairy Products

Butter and Margarine. People who are in the habit of spreading butter or margarine on breads, vegetables, and other foods can easily use up most of their daily fat budget by lunch time! The reason? Just one tablespoon of either of these products, in their full-fat versions, contains 11 grams of fat. If you add to this the butter and margarine used in cooking and baking, you can see the benefits of finding low- and no-fat alternatives.

How much fat can you save by using these substitute products? Reduced-fat margarine and light butter, which are made with less fat and more water, contain 33 to 80 percent less fat than full-fat versions. Products like Land O Lakes Light butter, I Can't Believe It's Not Butter! Light, Promise Light, Shedd's Spread Country Crock Light, and Mazola Light contain about half the fat of full-fat spreads. To cut fat by more than half, try a brand like Fleischmann's Lower Fat, Promise Ultra 70% Less Fat, Weight Watchers Light, or Smart Beat Lower-Fat. To eliminate fat completely, choose a fat-free product like I Can't Believe It's Not Butter! spray or tub margarine, Fleischmann's nonfat tub margarine, Fleischmann's nonfat squeeze margarine, and Promise Ultra Fat Free.

You may be surprised to find that you can also cook and bake with both reduced-fat margarine and light butter. Chapter 5 presents guidelines that will allow you to get delicious results whenever you substitute these products for their full-fat versions in cookies, cakes, muffins, and more.

Another fat-free alternative to butter and margarine is butter-flavored sprinkles. Made mostly of cornstarch with natural butter flavor, products like Butter Buds and Molly McButter come in handy shaker containers for sprinkling onto moist foods like baked potatoes and steamed vegetables. Butter Buds also comes in packets that can be mixed with water to make a pourable butter substitute.

Buttermilk. An essential ingredient in the low-fat kitchen, buttermilk adds a rich flavor and texture to all kinds of breads and baked goods, and lends a "cheesy" taste to sauces, dressings, and many other dishes. Originally a by-product of butter making, this product should perhaps be called "butterless" milk. Most brands of buttermilk are from 0.5 to 2 percent fat by weight, but some brands are as much as 3.5 percent fat. Choose brands that are no more than 1 percent milkfat. If you do not have buttermilk on hand, a good substitute can be made by mixing equal parts of nonfat yogurt and skim milk. Alternatively, place a tablespoon of vinegar or lemon juice in a one-cup measure, and fill to the one-cup mark with skim milk. Let the mixture sit for five minutes before using.

Milk. One gallon of whole milk contains 130 grams of fat—the equivalent of one and two thirds sticks of butter! And while you may not drink a gallon at a time, the fat you consume from milk can really add up. What are the best milk choices? Choose skim (nonfat) milk for the very least fat. Next in line is 1-percent low-fat or light milk, with about 2.5 grams ($^{1}/_{2}$ teaspoon) of fat per cup. What about 2-percent milk? Formerly called 2-percent low-fat milk, this product must now be called *reduced-fat* milk. The reason? By legal definition, a low-fat product can have no more than 3 grams of fat per serving. However, 2-percent milk contains 5 grams—a full teaspoon of butter—per cup. This labelling oversight has recently been corrected. Clearly, as the following table shows, skim and 1-percent milk are the better choices.

Calorie and Fat Comparison of Milks

Type of Milk (1-cup serving)	Calories	Fat
Whole milk (3.5% fat by weight)	150	8.0 g
2% reduced-fat milk (2% fat by weight)	130	5.0 g
1% low-fat or light milk (1% fat by weight)	100	2.5 g
Skim, fat-free, or nonfat milk (trace of fat)	90	0.5 g

People who cannot tolerate milk sugar—lactose—will be glad to know that most supermarkets stock Lactaid milk in a nonfat version. Nonfat Lactaid milk may be used in place of milk in any recipe. Some excellent nondairy alternatives to milk are also available. One tasty alternative is Rice Dream. This product, made from brown rice, has a creamy, slightly sweet taste that is similar to that of milk. Plain, unflavored Rice Dream is good for topping cereal and for cooking. Rice Dream is also available in several flavors. Whatever flavor you choose, be sure to get the 1-percent low-fat, calcium-fortified version. Several brands of low-fat calcium-fortified soymilk are also available in most grocery stores, and can be substituted for dairy milk in any recipe.

Sour Cream. As calorie- and fat-conscious people know, full-fat sour cream contains 48 grams of fat and almost 500 calories per cup! Use nonfat sour cream, though, and you'll eliminate at least half of the calories and all of the fat. Made from cultured non-fat milk thickened with vegetable gums, nonfat sour cream substitutes beautifully for its fatty counterpart in dips, spreads, sauces, and many other dishes. (See Chapter 5 for tips on using these nonfat products in your favorite recipes.)

Many brands of nonfat sour cream are available, including Land O Lakes No-Fat, Breakstone's Free, Sealtest Free, Guilt Free, and Naturally Yours No Fat. Most grocery store chains also sell their own brand of nonfat sour cream. Not ready to go totally fat-free with your sour cream yet? Many brands of reduced-fat and light sour cream are also available. These products contain half to a third less fat than full-fat brands, and are a nice start for people who are just beginning to get the fat out of their diets.

Yogurt. Plain nonfat or low-fat yogurt substitutes nicely for sour cream in cold dishes, dips, and dressings. And, as you will discover in Chapter 5, this product also adds creamy richness and flavor to sauces, baked goods, and casseroles and can even be made into a creamy cheese that can beautifully replace cream cheese in many dishes.

Flavored yogurts make a nutritious, calcium-rich snack. Of course, these yogurts do come packaged with varying amounts of fat and sugar—as much as 9 teaspoons of sugar and 1 1/2 teaspoons of fat per cup. While it is a simple matter to avoid unwanted fat in yogurt—just select one of the many nonfat or 1-percent brands—it is harder to determine how much added sugar is in a given container.

Why? The grams of sugar listed on the label include the naturally occurring milk sugar (lactose), plus any sugar present from added fruit, plus any added refined sugar. But if you keep in mind that one cup of plain yogurt contains about 16 grams of naturally occurring sugar, you can deduce that any sugar over this number has been added. For instance, if a cup of low-fat strawberry yogurt contains 46 grams of sugar, you can deduce that 30 of the grams come from added sugar (46 - 16 = 30). This is the equivalent of about 7 1/2 teaspoons of sugar (1 teaspoon of sugar = 4 grams). Some of the sugar is from the strawberries, but most is from a refined product.

To reduce your sugar intake, and therefore your calories, choose a plain unfla-vored yogurt, and then add your own fruit and just a couple of teaspoons of sugar or honey for sweetness. Or choose one of the many brands that are sweetened with aspartame, such as Dannon Light, Light n' Lively, Breyer's Light, La Yogur Light, and Weight Watchers Ultimate 90. These sugar-free brands contain 90 to 100 calories per cup—about half the calories of a sugar-sweetened yogurt. Realize, too, that yogurts come in both 6- and 8-ounce serving sizes, so the calories and sugar vary accordingly. And do be sure to select a brand that contains active yogurt cultures. Many brands display a seal on the label which indicates that the product meets National Yogurt Association standards for active cultures.

Nondairy Creamers and Whipped Toppings. Are nondairy coffee creamers and whipped toppings any better than the high-fat dairy products they are meant to replace? Sometimes. A glance at the ingredients list on most nondairy coffee creamers reveals them to be made of water, corn syrup, and partially hydrogenated vegetable oil—which contains cholesterol-raising trans-fatty acids. One tablespoon of these products provides about 20 calories and 1.5 grams of fat—about the same as that found in an equivalent amount of half-and-half. This makes full-fat nondairy creamers little better than cream. Fortunately, fat-free nondairy coffee creamers are available alongside the full-fat versions. With about 10 calories and 2 grams of sugar per tablespoon, these products are a better option than cream or half-and-half. Realize that the sweet, flavored versions are higher in calories. But for a truly healthy choice, try evaporated skimmed milk or instant nonfat dry milk powder, both of which will add nutrients to your coffee as they lighten it.

As for nondairy whipped toppings, the light versions—like Cool Whip Lite— contain about 80 percent less fat than whipped heavy cream, and half the fat of regular nondairy whipped toppings. Fat-free whipped toppings, such as Cool Whip Free and Kraft Free, are also available. With 15 calories and less than 0.5 gram of fat per serving, these products are a smart fat-fighting choice.

Eggs and Egg Substitutes

From breakfast omelettes and French toast to quiches, casseroles, and puddings, eggs are star ingredients in many foods. Most people know that eggs are also loaded with cholesterol—just one large egg uses up two thirds of your daily cholesterol budget. It also contains 5 grams of fat. This may not seem like all that much until you consider that a three-egg omelette contains 15 grams of fat—and that's without counting the cheese filling or the butter used in the skillet! The good news is that with the development of fat-free egg substitutes, you can now enjoy your favorite egg dishes with absolutely no fat or cholesterol at all.

Just what are egg substitutes? Contrary to what the term "substitute" implies, these products are made from 99 percent pure egg whites. The remaining 1 percent consists of vegetable thickeners and yellow coloring—usually beta-carotene or the plant-based coloring agents anatto or turmeric. You will find egg substitutes in both the refrigerated foods section and the freezer case. When selecting an egg substitute, look for fat-free brands like Egg Beaters, Better'n Eggs, Nulaid, Scramblers, and Second Nature. Many stores also have their own brand of fat-free egg substitute. Beware, though; a few brands contain vegetable oil, and so have almost as much fat as the eggs you are replacing.

THE MEAT COUNTER

Because of the high fat and cholesterol contents of meats, many people have sharply reduced their consumption of meat, have limited themselves to white meat chicken or turkey, or have totally eliminated meat and poultry from their diets. Happily, whether you are a sworn meat eater, someone who only occasionally eats meat dishes, or a confirmed vegetarian, plenty of lean meats, lean poultry, healthful seafood, and excellent meat substitutes are now available. The most important point to remember when including meat in meals is to keep portions to a modest six ounces or less per day. For perspective, three ounces of meat is the size of a deck of cards. Here are some suggestions for choosing the leanest possible poultry and meat.

Turkey

Although both chicken and turkey have less total fat and saturated fat than beef and pork, your very best bet when buying poultry is turkey. What's the difference between the fat and calorie contents of chicken and turkey? While 3 ounces of chicken breast without skin contain 139 calories and 3 grams of fat, the same amount of turkey breast without skin contains only 119 calories and 1 gram of fat.

All of the leanest cuts of turkey come from the breast, so that all have the same amount of fat and calories per serving. Below, you will learn about the cuts that you're likely to find at your local supermarket.

Turkey Cutlets. Turkey cutlets, which are slices of fresh turkey breast, are usually about 1/4-inch thick and weigh about 2 to 3 ounces each. These cutlets may be used as a delicious ultra-lean alternative to boneless chicken breast, pork tenderloin slices, or veal.

Turkey Medallions. Sliced from turkey tenderloins, medallions are about 1 inch thick and weigh about 2 to 3 ounces each. Turkey medallions can be substituted for pork or veal medallions.

Turkey Steaks. Cut from the turkey breast, these steaks are about 1/2 to 1 inch in thickness. Turkey steaks may be baked, broiled, grilled, cut into stir-fry pieces or kabobs, or ground for burgers.

Turkey Tenderloins. Large sections of fresh turkey breast, tenderloins usually weigh about 8 ounces each. Tenderloins may be sliced into cutlets, cut into stir-fry or kabob pieces, ground for burgers, or grilled or roasted as is.

Whole Turkey Breasts. Perfect for people who love roast turkey but want only the breast meat, turkey breasts weigh 4 to 8 pounds each. These breasts may be roasted with or without stuffing.

Ground Turkey. Ground turkey is an excellent ingredient for use in meatballs, chili, burgers—in any dish that uses ground meat. When shopping for ground turkey, though, you'll find that different products have different percentages of fat, and unless you read labels, you may get more than you bargained for. Your very leanest choice is ground turkey breast, and many brands are now widely available. These products

The Skinny on Skinning Poultry

Most people know that one of the best ways to trim the fat from poultry is to remove the skin. By removing the skin and any underlying visible fat, you eliminate over half the fat. Is there any advantage to removing the skin *before* cooking? A slight one. Poultry cooked without the skin has about 20 percent less fat than poultry whose skin is removed after cooking. This amounts to about 1.5 grams of fat saved by removing the skin from a chicken breast before cooking instead of after. Also, when the skin is removed after cooking, the seasoning is, too—another reason to take off that skin before you start preparing your dish.

will be between 97- and 99-percent lean and contain 1 to 3 grams of fat per 3.5-ounce cooked serving. Next in line are mixtures that contain skinless dark meat, which will be about 95-percent lean and provide 4 to 5 grams of fat per serving. In contrast, brands that provide no nutrition information are typically made with added skin and fat. These products may contain over 15 percent fat by weight and 12 to 17 grams of fat per serving. This is more fat than you'll find in many kinds of ground beef! The moral is clear. Always check labels before making a purchase.

Chicken

Though not as low in fat as turkey, chicken is still lower in fat than most cuts of beef and pork, and therefore is a valuable ingredient in low-fat cooking. Beware, though: many cuts of chicken, if eaten with the skin on, contain more fat than some cuts of beef and pork. For the least fat, choose the chicken breast and always remove the skin—preferably, before cooking.

Comparing Chicken Parts

Part (3-ounce cooked portion)	Calories	Fat
Breast, with skin	167	6.6 g
Breast, skin removed before cooking	125	1.4 g
Breast, skin removed after cooking	139	3.0 g
Leg, with skin	183	9.5 g
Leg, without skin	146	4.8 g
Thigh, with skin	210	13.2 g
Thigh, without skin	178	9.3 g
Wing, with skin	247	16.6 g
Wing, without skin	173	6.9 g

Where does ground chicken fit in? Like ground turkey, ground chicken often contains skin and fat. In fact, most brands contain at least 15 percent fat, so read the labels before you buy.

Beef and Pork

Although not as lean as turkey, beef and pork are both considerably leaner today than in decades past. Spurred by competition from the poultry industry, beef and pork producers have changed breeding and feeding practices to reduce the fat content of these products. In addition, butchers are now trimming away more of the fat from retail cuts of meat. The result? On average, grocery store cuts of beef are 27 percent leaner today than they were in the early 1980s, and retail cuts of pork are 43 percent leaner.

Of course, some cuts of beef and pork are leaner than others. Which are the smartest choices? The following table will guide you in selecting those cuts of beef and pork that are lowest in fat.

The Leanest Beef and Pork Cuts

Part (3-ounce cooked portion)	Calories	Fat
Beef		
Eye of Round	143	4.2 g
Top Round	153	4.2 g
Round Tip	157	5.9 g
Top Sirloin	165	6.1 g
Pork		
Tenderloin	139	4.1 g
Ham (95% lean)	112	4.3 g
Boneless Sirloin Chops	164	5.7 g
Boneless Loin Roast	165	6.1 g
Boneless Loin Chops	173	6.6 g

While identifying the lowest-fat cuts of meat is an important first step in healthy cooking, be aware that even lean cuts have varying amounts of fat because of differences in grades. In general, the higher and more expensive grades of meat, like USDA Prime and Choice, have more fat due to a higher degree of marbling—internal fat that cannot be trimmed away. USDA Select meats have the least amount of marbling, and therefore the lowest amount of fat. How important are these differences? A USDA Choice piece of meat may have 15 to 20 percent more fat than a USDA Select cut, and USDA Prime may have even more fat. Clearly, the difference is significant. So when choosing beef and pork for your table, by all means check the package for grade. Then look for the least amount of marbling in the cut you have chosen, and let appearance be your final guide.

Ground Beef. No food adds more fat—and, most especially, saturated fat—to people's diets than ground beef. Just how fatty is ground beef? At its worst, it is almost 33 percent pure fat. And ground sirloin and round are not necessarily leaner. Terms like sirloin and round merely indicate the part of the animal from which the meat came, not the amount of fat it contains.

The only way to be sure of fat content is to buy meat whose label provides some nutrition information. However, if your only choices are unlabelled packages of ground beef, choose the type that is darkest in color. As the fat content goes up, the color of ground beef becomes paler.

To obtain the leanest ground beef possible, you can select a piece of top round and have the butcher trim and grind it for you. Ground beef made this way has about 132 calories and 4.9 grams of fat per 3-ounce cooked serving, and is about 95-percent lean. Most stores also carry prepackaged ground beef that is 93-percent lean. This is also an acceptable choice. In fact, you may be surprised to learn that 93-percent lean ground beef contains about half the fat of most ground turkey—which is about 85-percent lean—making the beef a better choice in this case. (Of course, 97- to 99-percent lean ground turkey is still the leanest choice of all.) The following table, which compares different grinds of beef, shows that as the percentage of fat decreases, so do the calorie and fat-gram counts.

Comparing Ground Beef

Grind (3-ounce cooked portion)	Calories	Fat
73% lean (27% fat by weight)	248	17.9 g
80% lean (20% fat by weight)	228	15.2 g
85% lean (15% fat by weight)	204	12.2 g
90% lean (10% fat by weight)	169	9.1 g
93% lean (7% fat by weight)	134	6.0 g
95% lean (5% fat by weight)	132	4.9 g

If you are not used to cooking with meat that is as lean as 95-percent lean ground meat, you may be surprised to find that there is no fat to drain. In fact, the beef may stick to the bottom of the pan during browning. If this happens, simply add a few tablespoons of water to the skillet.

Lean Processed Meats

Because of our new fat-consciousness, low-fat bacon, ham, hot dogs, lunchmeats, and sausages are now available, with just a fraction of the fat of regular processed meats. Here are some examples.

Bacon. Turkey bacon, made with strips of light and dark turkey meat, looks and tastes much like pork bacon. But with 30 calories and 0.5 to 2 grams of fat per strip, turkey bacon has 50 percent less fat than crisp-cooked pork bacon, and shrinks much less during cooking. Besides being a leaner alternative to regular breakfast bacon, turkey bacon may be substituted for pork bacon in Southern-style vegetables, casseroles, and other dishes. Look for brands like Butterball, Louis Rich, Mr. Turkey, and Jennie-O.

Canadian bacon, which has always been about 95-percent lean, is another useful ingredient in the low-fat kitchen. Use this flavorful product in breakfast casseroles and soups, and as a topping for pizzas.

Ham. Low-fat hams are made from either pork or turkey. These products contain as little as 0.5 gram of fat per ounce. Of course, all cured hams, including the leaner brands, are very high in sodium. However, used in moderation—to flavor bean soups or breakfast casseroles, for instance—these products can be incorporated into a healthy diet. Just avoid adding further salt to your recipes. Look for brands like Healthy Choice hams, Hormel Curemaster 96% fat-free ham, Butterball turkey ham, Hormel Light & Lean ham, and Boar's Head lean hams.

Hot Dogs. When most people think of lighter hot dogs, turkey franks immediately come to mind. True, turkey franks do contain 30 to 50 percent less fat than regular hot dogs, but most brands still contain about 8 grams—2 teaspoons—of fat each. Fortunately, some very low-fat and fat-free brands of hot dogs are also available. Oscar Mayer Free, Bryan Fat-Free, Butterball Free, Ball Park Fat-Free, and Hormel Light & Lean hot dogs are all good options. All of these dogs are fat-free, and therefore save you 16 grams of fat compared with regular franks. Healthy Choice hot dogs are another very low-fat option. As with all hot dogs, sodium is still a problem, so use these products in moderation.

Lunchmeats. Many brands of ultra-lean lunchmeats are now available, including Healthy Choice, Butterball, Louis Rich, Mr. Turkey, Oscar Mayer Free, and many varieties of Boar's Head. Today's low-fat deli meats include everything from pastrami and corned beef to bologna, roast beef, turkey, and ham. These meats make ideal substitutes for fatty cold cuts in sandwiches and party platters. Like all processed meats, though, they should be used in moderation due to their high sodium content.

Some processed meats are now labelled "fat-free." Since all meats naturally contain some fat, how can this be? The manufacturer first starts with a lean meat such as turkey breast, and then adds enough water to dilute the fat to a point where the product contains less than 0.5 gram of fat per serving. Fortunately, meats that are labelled 96- to 99-percent lean—and therefore contain 0.3 to 1 gram of fat per ounce—are also lean enough to be included in a low-fat diet.

Sausage. A variety of low-fat and fat-free sausages made from turkey, or a combination of turkey, beef, and pork, is now available. These products contain a mere 30 to 40 calories and less than 0.5 to 3 grams of fat per ounce. Compare this with an ounce of full-fat pork sausage, which contains over 100 calories and almost 9 grams of fat, and you'll see what a boon these new healthier mixtures are. Beware, though: While labelled "light," some brands of sausage contain as much as 14 grams of fat per 2.5-ounce serving. This is half the amount of fat found in the same-size serving of regular pork sausage, but is still a hefty dose of fat for such a small portion of food.

When a recipe calls for smoked turkey or kielbasa sausage, try a fat-free brand like Butterball Fat Free. Or use Healthy Choice or Hillshire Farm 97% Fat-Free, both of which have less than 1 gram of fat per ounce. Louis Rich and Mr. Turkey are other good reduced-fat brands. When buying bulk ground turkey breakfast sausage, try brands like Louis Rich, which contains 75 percent less fat than ground pork sausage. Many stores also make their own fresh turkey sausage, including turkey Italian sausage. When buying fresh sausage, always check the package labels and choose the leanest mixture available.

Vegetarian Alternatives

Nonmeat alternatives to ground meat, sausage, and other meat products are now wide-ly available in grocery stores. One product you will find in the produce section of most stores is Marjon Tofu Crumbles. These precooked, mildly seasoned, textured bits of tofu are a great low-fat substitute for all or part of the ground meat in chili, sloppy Joes, tacos, and other dishes. Two other ground meat substitutes that you will find in the freezer case are Morningstar Farms ground meatless and Green Giant Harvest Burger for Recipes. Made from soybeans and other vegetable proteins, these fat-free products look and taste much like cooked crumbled ground beef. Another great ground meat alternative is texturized vegetable protein (TVP). Made from defat-ted soybean flour that has been formed into small nuggets, this product is fat- and cho-lesterol-free, rich in protein, and very economical. TVP is widely available in health foods stores and some grocery stores. Like tofu crumbles and ground meatless crum-bles, TVP can replace all or part of the ground meat in many dishes. Chapter 5 will show you how to use these products in your favorite recipes.

Your freezer case offers still more alternatives to meat. Looking for a ready-made meatless burger? Try Green Giant Harvest Burgers, Wholesome & Hearty Garden-Burgers, or Morningstar Farms Better'n Burgers, all of which can also be found in the freezer case of many grocery stores. With just a fraction of the fat of their ground beef counterparts, these tasty burgers also provide some fiber.

Nonmeat breakfast alternatives are also available. Choose from Wholesome & Hearty Garden-Sausage, with only 1 gram of fat per ounce; Morningstar Farms Breakfast Links, with 82 percent less fat than pork links; and many others. (Again, these can be found in the freezer case.) Do read labels, though. Just because a food is vegetarian, does not necessarily mean it is low in fat. In fact, some meat alternatives contain just as much fat as the meat they are meant to replace.

Fish and Other Seafood

Of the many kinds of fish and other seafood now available, some is almost fat-free, while some is moderately fatty. However, the oil in fish provides an essential kind of fat—known as omega-3 fatty acids—that most people's diets do not supply in suffi-cient quantities. The omega-3 fats in fish can help reduce blood triglycerides, lower blood pressure, prevent the formation of deadly blood clots, and provide many other health benefits. This means that all kinds of fish—including the more oily ones like salmon, mackerel, mullet, and sardines—are considered healthful. In fact, eating just two meals of fish a week can help prevent heart disease.

Many commercial fish are now raised on "farms." Do these fish offer the same health benefits as fish that are caught in natural habitats? No. Farm-raised fish are fed grains instead of their natural diet of plankton and smaller fish. As a result, these fish contain as much or more fat than wild fish, but are much lower in the beneficial omega-3 fats.

What about the cholesterol content of shellfish? It may not be as high as you think it is. With the exception of shrimp and oysters, a 3-ounce serving of most shellfish has about 60 milligrams of cholesterol—well under the daily upper limit of 300 milligrams. The same-size serving of shrimp has about 166 milligrams of cholesterol, which is just over half the recommended daily limit. Oysters have about 90 milligrams of cholesterol. However, all seafood, including shellfish, is very low in saturated fat, which has a greater cholesterol-raising effect than does cholesterol. The following table, which compares several common fish and shellfish, should help you stay within your daily calorie, fat, and cholesterol budgets.

Comparing Seafood

Seafood (3-ounce cooked portion)	Calories	Fat	Cholesterol
Clams	126	1.7 g	57 mg
Crab, Alaskan King	82	1.3 g	45 mg
Flounder	99	1.3 g	58 mg
Grouper	100	1.1 g	40 mg
Haddock	95	0.8 g	63 mg
Halibut	119	2.5 g	35 mg
Lobster	83	0.5 g	61 mg
Mackerel, Spanish	134	5.4 g	62 mg
Mullet	127	4.1 g	54 mg
Mussels	147	3.8 g	48 mg
Oysters	117	4.2 g	89 mg
Pollock	96	1.0 g	82 mg
Salmon, Coho	157	6.4 g	42 mg
Sardines (not oil packed)	151	10.2 g	52 mg
Scallops	113	3.3 g	34 mg
Shrimp	84	0.9 g	166 mg
Sole	99	1.3 g	58 mg
Swordfish	132	4.4 g	43 mg

Fish is highly perishable, so it is important to know how to select a high-quality product. First, make sure that the fish is firm and springy to the touch. Second, buy fish only if it has a clean seaweed odor, rather than a "fishy" smell. Third, when purchasing whole fish, choose those fish whose gills are bright red in color, and whose eyes are clear and bulging, not sunken or cloudy. Finally refrigerate fish as soon as you get it home, and be sure to cook it within forty-eight hours of purchase.

OILS

Like butter and margarine, oils used in cooking, baking, and salad dressings can blow your fat budget in a hurry. Many people are confused about oils because liquid vegetable oils have long been promoted as being "heart healthy." The reason? These oils are low in artery-clogging saturated fat, and contain no cholesterol. Unfortunately, many people also assume that these products are low in total fat and calories, and therefore may be used liberally. Not so. The fact is that all oils are pure fat. Just one tablespoon of *any* oil has 13.6 grams of fat and 120 calories. Vegetable oils do provide the essential fats that are needed for good health, but so do plenty of other foods, such as vegetables, whole grains, fish, nuts, and seeds. A well-balanced diet that includes these foods can provide more than enough essential fat—without the addition of *any* vegetable oil. However, sometimes a recipe does require a small amount of vegetable oil, and used sparingly, these products can be part of a low-fat diet.

Which vegetable oils are best? Those that are low in saturated fats and rich in monounsaturated fats—like olive and canola oil—are the oils of choice these days. However, if you keep your use of all fats and oils to a minimum, any liquid vegetable oil, depending on your taste and cooking preferences, is fine. Some vegetable oils, though, are more useful to the low-fat cook than others. Here are a few products you might consider buying on your next trip to the grocery store.

Canola Oil. This has become one of the oils of choice in recent years. Low in saturated fats and rich in monounsaturated fats, canola oil also contains a fair amount of linolenic acid, an essential omega-3 type fat—similar to the fat found in fish oils—that most people do not eat in sufficient quantities. Canola oil has a very mild, bland taste, so it is a good all-purpose oil for cooking and baking when you want no interfering flavors. Like all oils, this product should be used sparingly to keep calories under control.

Extra Virgin Olive Oil. Unlike most vegetable oils, which are very bland, olive oil adds its own delicious flavor to foods. Extra virgin olive oil is the least processed and most flavorful type of olive oil. And a little bit goes a long way, making this product a good choice for use in low-fat recipes. What about "light" olive oil? In this case, light refers to flavor, which is mild and bland compared with that of extra virgin oils. This means that you have to use more oil for the same amount of flavor—not a good bargain.

Macadamia Nut Oil. Like olive and canola oils, macadamia nut oil is low in saturated fats and rich in monounsaturated fats. And like canola oil, macadamia nut oil contains a fair amount of linolenic acid. An excellent all-purpose oil for cooking and baking, this product adds a delicate nutty flavor to foods.

Sesame Oil. Like olive oil, sesame oil can enhance the flavors of foods. In small amounts, this ingredient will add a distinctive taste to foods without blowing your fat budget.

Unrefined Corn Oil. Most of the vegetable oils sold in grocery stores today have been highly processed and refined, greatly extending their shelf life. Unfortunately, processing also depletes oils of much of their natural nutty flavor and aroma—and of close to half of their vitamin E content. Most people grew up on these comparatively bland, tasteless refined oils, and have never even seen an unprocessed vegetable oil. They don't know what they're missing. Many stores stock at least one brand of unrefined oil, such as the widely available Spectrum unrefined corn oil. This amber-colored, buttery tasting oil is excellent for baking. And because it is so flavorful, a small amount is all you'll need in your low-fat recipes. Once opened, unrefined oils can turn rancid quickly. For this reason, you should purchase small bottles—a pint or less—and store the oil in the refrigerator.

Walnut Oil. With a delicate nutty flavor, walnut oil is another excellent choice for baking and cooking. This oil also contains a fair amount of the omega-3 fat linolenic acid. Most brands of walnut oil have been only minimally processed, so like unrefined corn oil, this oil should be kept in the refrigerator.

Nonstick Vegetable Oil Cooking Spray. Available unflavored and in butter and olive oil flavors, these products are pure fat. The advantage to using them is that the amount that comes out during a one-second spray is so small that it adds an insignificant amount of fat to a recipe. Nonstick cooking sprays are very useful to the low-fat cook to promote the browning of foods and to prevent foods from sticking to pots and pans. Look for products like PAM Butter Flavor No Stick Cooking Spray, PAM Olive Oil No Stick Cooking Spray, Mazola No Stick cooking spray, and Wesson No Stick cooking spray. When a recipe directs you to both grease and flour a pan, use Baker's Joy spray, which combines oil and flour in one handy product.

BREAD

Bread really is the staff of life. If you don't believe it, just consider the Food Guide Pyramid created by the U.S. Department of Agriculture. Bread and other grain products form the base of this guide to dietary choices, with at least six servings of these products recommended daily. But all bread is not created equal. Let's take a look at some of the factors you'll want to consider when buying bread for your family.

Fat

Bread is often thought of as a "fattening" food. But the fact is that most breads—including sandwich breads, pita bread, bagels, and English muffins—contain only 80 calories and 1 gram of fat per slice. Choose a biscuit or croissant, though, and the extra fat can cause the calorie count to more than double. As for muffins and quick breads, many contain far too much fat and sugar. And don't be fooled by fat-free muffins. Many are as nutritionally poor as a fat-free cupcake, and contain comparable amounts of sugar and calories. Always read labels to be sure of what you are getting.

White Versus Whole Wheat

Whole wheat bread, which is made with the entire wheat kernel, is far better than white bread. Why? Whole wheat bread's superior fiber count is one reason. Breads made from 100-percent whole wheat flour provide 4 to 5 grams of fiber for each two-slice serving, while the same-size serving of white bread contains only a gram. Whole grain breads also provide a wealth of nutrients such as vitamins B_6 and E, folate, copper, zinc, iron, chromium, manganese, and magnesium—nutrients that have been processed out of white bread.

How do you know if a bread is whole grain? Look at the ingredients list. Whole wheat flour or another whole grain should be the first ingredient listed. Be aware that some breads, although bearing names like "natural wheat" and "honey wheat," contain very little whole wheat flour. Instead, they are made with "wheat flour" or "unbleached wheat flour"—both of which refer to refined white flour. Where do rye and pumpernickel breads fit in? These breads typically contain far more white flour than they do whole grains. Nutritionally, they will fall somewhere between white bread and 100-percent whole wheat bread.

Light Versus Regular Bread

In "light" breads, indigestible plant fibers replace part of the flour. Because these fibers cannot be digested, breads made with these ingredients have half the calories of regular breads. How does light bread compare with 100-percent whole grain bread? Most light breads contain as much or more fiber than whole grain breads do. However, most are also made with refined wheat flour, and so do not provide the same nutrients as 100-percent whole grain bread. If you prefer light bread, you will get the most nutritional value by choosing a brand that lists whole wheat flour as the first ingredient.

Sodium

Over the course of a day, bread can contribute a surprising amount of sodium to your diet, with most breads providing 130 to 175 milligrams of sodium per slice. And pumpernickel, rye bread, biscuits, and quick breads tend to contain twice as much sodium as whole wheat and white breads. To keep your sodium intake under control, look for breads that contain no more than 150 milligrams per slice.

Some Breads to Put in Your Basket

Since most breads are low in fat, it is impossible to list all of the many brands from which you can choose. However, a few brands are noteworthy for their excellent nutritional value.

Fiber-Rich Whole Grain Breads

Among the best choices are Arnold Bran'nola Dark Wheat, Arnold Stoneground 100% Whole Wheat, Country Farms 100% Whole Wheat, Nature's Own 100% Whole

Wheat, Grant's Farm 100% Whole Wheat, Oroweat Light 100% Whole Wheat, Pepperidge Farm 100% Stoneground Whole Wheat, Pepperidge Farm Natural Whole Grain Crunchy Grains, Roman Meal 100% Whole Wheat, and most brands labelled "100% Whole Wheat." In addition, Matthew's and Brownberry each offer a fine selection of preservative-free whole grain breads.

Part Whole Grain Breads

Oatmeal, rye, pumpernickel, and mixed grain breads are also acceptable choices, since they contain at least some whole grain flour. As previously mentioned, they also tend to be rather high in sodium. Two good products—ones that are relatively low in sodium—are Arnold Pumpernickel and Merita New York Soft Rye.

Other Healthful Choices

For a change of pace, try whole grain English muffins, whole grain bagels, and whole wheat or oat bran pita bread. Tortillas made from corn and whole wheat flour are other good choices. French bread, sourdough bread, white flour tortillas, and many other specialty breads are other low-fat options, though they do not provide the fiber and nutrients that whole grain breads do.

CEREALS AND OTHER BREAKFAST FOODS

Breakfast is truly the most important meal of the day. Besides giving your metabolism a boost, breakfast—if chosen wisely—can be quick, easy, supernutritious, and practically fat-free. Let's take a look at some products you may want to stock up on, as well as some you may wish to avoid, during your next trip to the grocery store.

Cereals

Breakfast just doesn't get any easier than a bowl of cereal. And if you choose the right cereal, breakfast can be quick to prepare and nutritious. Fiber, complex carbohydrates, and B vitamins are just a few of the nutrients that a morning bowl of cereal can provide.

The first rule of buying cereal is this: Don't look down—to the lower shelves in the grocery store, that is. Quite often, the lower shelves, which are at a child's eye level, feature the sugary refined products that are meant to appeal to kids. The more nutritious choices tend to fill the store's upper shelves. How can you tell which cereals are best? Choose brands that are low in added fats and sugars and high in whole grains and fiber. Use the following guidelines to evaluate cereals.

Fat

When selecting a cereal, keep in mind that most are quite low in fat. Old-fashioned granola is an exception to this rule, but these days, several brands of delicious low-fat and fat-free granolas are widely available. And don't automatically reject a cereal just because it contains a couple of grams of fat. The fact is that most whole grain cereals do contain some fat per serving because whole grains include the wholesome germ—the inner portion of the grain that is an important source of essential fatty acids, vitamin E, and other nutrients. While some refined cereals may be lower in fat, nutri-

Top Choice Cereals

When chosen wisely, breakfast cereals can provide both great taste and great nutrition. The Best Bets in the first list are all 100-percent whole grain cereals, with no added sugar, salt, or fat. These are my number-one recommendations. The products in the second list, though, are also noteworthy—100-percent whole grain cereals, with low to moderate amounts of sugar and no added fat. Note that any product followed by an asterisk (*) is sweetened with fruit juice instead of refined sugar, and so is a particularly good choice.

Best Bets

☐ Nabisco Shredded Wheat
☐ Plain oatmeal or oat bran
☐ Puffed whole grain cereals like
   Arrowhead Mills Puffed Wheat
   and Puffed Kamut
☐ Quaker Multigrain Oatmeal
☐ Ralston hot cereal
☐ Wheatena hot cereal

Other Good Choices

☐ Arrowhead Mills cereals*
☐ Dr. McDougall's Right Foods
   instant oatmeals
☐ General Mills Cheerios
☐ General Mills Fiber One

☐ General Mills Total
☐ General Mills Wheaties
☐ Health Valley cereals*
☐ Kellogg's All-Bran
☐ Kellogg's Common Sense
   Oat Bran flakes
☐ Kellogg's Just Right
☐ Kellogg's Nutrigrain
☐ Nabisco 100% Bran
☐ Post Grape-Nuts
☐ Post Natural Bran Flakes
☐ Quaker Oat Life
☐ Quaker Oat Squares
☐ Ralston Wheat Chex
☐ Ralston Multibran Chex
☐ Uncle Sam Cereal

tionally, they do not compare to whole grain products. Nuts can also contribute fat to cereals. But the oil in nuts, like that in whole grains, provides essential nutrients along with the fat. What you want to avoid is a cereal with added fat, like partially hydrogenated vegetable oil, which will be listed in the ingredients list. As a general rule, try to keep the fat count per serving down to 3 grams.

Fiber

Look at the ingredients list. A whole grain should be listed as the first—and, therefore, the main—ingredient. Whole grain cereals provide at least 4 grams of fiber per 2-ounce serving—unless, of course, they're puffed, like whole grain puffed wheat. Cereals that contain added bran provide even more fiber.

Sugar

Look at the Nutrition Facts label to see how much sugar your cereal contains. Four grams of sugar is the equivalent of 1 teaspoon of sugar, so that a cereal with 12 grams per serving provides 3 teaspoons of sugar. The picture is not as clear, though, when cereals contain added fruit, because the label groups the fruit's sugar with the cereal's added refined sugar. Compare the amount of sugar in your cereal with a prudent daily limit of 40 to 50 grams (about 10 to 12^1/$_2$ teaspoons), and you will see how your cereal fits into your diet.

When scanning your supermarket's shelves, don't overlook store brands. Compare the Nutrition Facts labels and ingredients lists, and you will see that many store brands are practically identical to national brands, but are a better value.

You may be surprised that cereals like Rice Krispies, Special K, corn flakes, and Cream of Wheat are not among the highly recommended cereals. Why? Though these cereals are low in fat and sugar, they are made from refined grains, and therefore contain little or no fiber and lack many nutrients compared with whole grain cereals.

Cereal Bars and Toaster Pastries

Also located in the cereal aisle is a large selection of low-fat and fat-free cereal bars, breakfast bars, and toaster pastries. Advertised as being "wholesome" or "made with real fruit and grains," these products are often assumed to be a good alternative to a bowl of cereal. Just how nutritious are they? Not very. A glance at the Nutrition Facts label and the ingredients list reveals that the typical cereal bar contains about 4 teaspoons of sugar and only 1 gram of fiber. Refined carbohydrates like white flour and sugar top the list of ingredients. And though these bars are made with fruit, the amount is so small as to be insignificant.

As for toaster pastries, like cereal bars, these products are combinations of refined flour and sugar. Since toaster pastries tend to be larger than cereal bars, they will contain about 5 teaspoons of sugar apiece. Healthy exceptions in the breakfast bar category include Health Valley's Fat-Free Cereal Bars and Healthy Tarts, and Jammers toaster pastries. Made with 100 percent whole wheat flour and sweetened with real fruits, these products provide 3 grams of fiber and plenty of nutrients.

Pancake Mixes

Pancakes are a favorite weekend breakfast treat in many households, and to save time, some people prefer to use a mix. How nutritious are pancake mixes? With a few exceptions, not as nutritious as you might think. Most major brands of pancake and waffle mixes are made from refined flours, and so provide no fiber and few nutrients. Two exceptions are Hodgson Mill and Arrowhead Mills whole grain pancake mixes. Both manufacturers offer a variety of pancake mixes made with wholesome whole grain flours. Aunt Jemima Buckwheat pancake mix is also made with whole grain buckwheat flour. One serving—four pancakes—supplies a respectable 4 grams of fiber. And if you leave out the oil using the guidelines on page 79, and use an egg substitute or egg whites when mixing up the batter, your cakes will be practically fat-free.

Light and reduced-calorie pancake mixes also supply some fiber from added cellulose—a refined fiber used as a bulking agent in reduced-calorie baked goods. But since these products are still made mostly of white flour, nutritionally speaking, you will be better off with a whole grain product.

Fortunately, pancakes are almost as simple to make from scratch as they are from a mix. Try making your favorite pancake recipe substituting whole wheat flour or oats for part of the refined flour. Then replace the oil in the recipe as described on page 79, and your pancakes will be as nutritious as they are delicious.

CANNED GOODS

No one can dispute the convenience of canned foods. It is true, though, that canned foods tend to be very salty. In fact, a one-pound can of vegetables often contains up to a teaspoon of salt—nearly a full-day's allowance of sodium. But many manufacturers are now producing reduced-salt and unsalted products that work beautifully in a healthy low-fat, low-sodium diet.

How do canned foods compare with fresh nutritionally? In general, fresh and frozen foods retain more nutritional value than do canned foods. The reason? The heating process required for canning foods destroys some nutrients, including vitamin C and the B vitamin folate. In addition, minerals like potassium and the B vitamins leach into the canning liquid. If you pour off the canning liquid in an effort to reduce the salt, you will also lose some of these nutrients.

However, it may surprise you to learn that canned foods are sometimes *more* nutritious than fresh. How can this be? Properly canned foods are picked at their peak of ripeness and then quickly processed. Produce that is destined to be sold fresh, however, is often picked slightly underripe, transported across the country, and then left to sit in storage for as much as several days before being purchased. Once you get the food home, it may then sit in the refrigerator for several days more before you eat it. If this is the case, you could be better off with a canned product—although frozen produce would be an even better choice. The rest of this section describes some canned foods worth stocking in your pantry.

Beans. Canned beans are another good item to have on hand. Full of fiber and nutrients, canned garbanzos, kidney beans, black beans, and the many other varieties now available make wonderful additions to soups, salads, and casseroles. If you drain and rinse the beans before adding them to your recipe, you will reduce the sodium by about 40 percent. Or try Eden canned beans, which are grown organically and processed without salt.

Evaporated Skimmed Milk. Another must for your low-fat pantry is evaporated skimmed milk, which is a wonderfully versatile ingredient that can be substituted for cream in many dishes. Try brands like Carnation Fat Free and Pet, which are both widely available.

Fruits. Fruits packed in juice, such as Libby's Lite and Del Monte Lite; unsweetened applesauce; and crushed pineapple in juice, are also good canned food choices. Enjoy them as snacks, or use them in any number of recipes.

Low-Sugar Pie Fillings. Light (reduced-sugar) pie fillings—like Comstock Light and Lucky Leaf Lite—are also nice to keep on hand. These products make a tasty topping for waffles or pancakes, and contain a lot less sugar than syrup.

Meats. Water-packed canned tuna, chicken, and turkey are other worthwhile pantry staples. Keep these ingredients on hand for making salads, sandwiches, and casseroles.

Pasta Sauces. Canned and bottled fat-free and low-fat pasta sauces enable the fat-fighting cook to prepare tasty, nutritious meals in a matter of minutes. Read more about these products on page 57.

Soups. Several brands of reduced-sodium, low-fat soups are available for those times when you need a meal in a matter of minutes. Read more about these products on page 56.

Tomato Products. Unsalted canned tomato products—like Hunt's No Salt Added tomatoes, tomato sauce, and tomato paste; Eden crushed tomatoes and tomato sauce; Cento crushed tomatoes; and Del Monte No Salt Added stewed tomatoes—are excellent choices for your pantry. Progresso Recipe Ready crushed tomatoes with added purée is another handy ingredient that contains far less sodium than most brands of canned tomatoes. Use these products in your soups, chilies, pasta sauces, and countless other dishes.

FRUIT JUICES

Whether fresh, canned, bottled, or frozen, fruit juices are often enjoyed as a refreshing alternative to sugary sodas. And since juices are naturally fat-free, people often assume they can drink unlimited quantities. Beware, though, if you are watching your weight, as fruit juices contain just as much—and sometimes more—calories than sodas do. People who use juices to quench their thirst instead of water may be taking in a lot more calories than they realize. Furthermore, what many people think of as juice is actually fruit-flavored sugar water. How can you tell the difference? Read labels, and look for beverages that state they are "100 percent juice." Another tip-off is the name of the drink. If a drink is called "fruit punch," "fruit cooler," "fruit ade," "fruit juice cocktail," or "fruit beverage," take a look at the ingredients list. The beverage will most likely be a combination of sugar, water, and artificial flavors mixed with little or no real fruit juice.

How do fruit juices stack up to whole fruits? Not very well. Juices contain none of the fiber that is naturally present in whole fruits. For this reason, drinking a glass of juice is not as filling and satisfying as eating a piece of fruit would be. And once exposed to air, juices can quickly lose nutrients like vitamin C and folate. In contrast, these nutrients remain well preserved inside a piece of fresh fruit.

What about the sports drinks that are often sold alongside juices? These beverages are simply mixtures of refined sugar, water, potassium, and salt that are sold at a premium price. One quart of most sports drinks will provide about 15 teaspoons of sugar, 1/5 teaspoon of salt, and less potassium than you will get in a quarter of a banana. Since most people get more than enough carbohydrate and salt in their daily diets, these drinks are generally of no value. And if you are exercising in an effort to lose weight, consuming large amounts of sports beverages can slow your progress. For instance, a one-hour aerobics class or an hour spent mowing the lawn will burn about 450 calories. If you drink a quart of sports beverage during your activity, you will consume about 240 calories, largely offsetting your efforts. Being properly hydrated is crucial during exercise, but plain water works perfectly well. Just drink plenty before, during, and after exercise. As for sodium and potassium, in all but extreme cases, these minerals can easily be replaced by eating a well-balanced diet.

SOUPS, BROTHS, AND BOUILLONS

It's hard to find a quicker or easier meal than canned soup. But until recently, you often had to sacrifice nutrition for the sake of convenience. Fortunately, those days have passed. Several manufacturers now offer entire lines of no- and low-fat soups that contain 30 to 50 percent less sodium than traditional canned soups. Also available is a variety of low-sodium bouillons—a boon to the health-conscious cook who simply doesn't have time to prepare a homemade stock. Let's take a look at some of the products that may be available at your local grocery or health foods store.

Canned Soups and Broths. Looking for a tasty low-fat, low-sodium soup to accompany your lunch-time sandwich? Nowadays, your choices are greater than ever before. Look for brands like Campbell's Healthy Request, Hain Naturals Low Fat and 99% Fat Free, Health Valley, Healthy Choice, Progresso 99% Fat Free, and Pritikin. For a hearty soup that is loaded with cholesterol-lowering soluble fiber, try bean, split pea, or lentil soup. To get your five-a-day of vegetables, choose a hearty tomato or vegetable soup. And if it's calcium you're looking for, choose a soup that's prepared with milk—and then use nonfat or 1-percent milk.

Every cook knows that canned soups are not only great-tasting dishes in themselves, but also wonderful ingredients in all kinds of recipes. Looking for a low-fat cream of mushroom or cream of celery soup to add to your favorite casserole? Try Campbell's Healthy Request. And for a convenient broth to serve as a base for your own homemade soups, look for brands like Campbell's Healthy Request, Swanson Natural Goodness, and Health Valley No Salt Added chicken broths. Health Valley also makes a fat-free, low-sodium beef broth, and Swanson and Hain both make low-fat vegetable broths.

Dry Bouillons and Bases. Dry bouillons, like canned soups, are great to have on hand for those days when there's no time to make soup stock from scratch. Available in beef, chicken, ham, vegetable, and onion flavors, bouillons can also add flavor to vegetable side dishes, casseroles, and many other culinary creations.

The good news is that most bouillons are fat-free. The bad news is that most contain a whopping 1,000 milligrams of sodium per teaspoon. Maggi instant bouillon granules and Wyler's reduced sodium bouillons, both widely available products, contain about 30-percent less sodium than the average bouillon. Also available are very low-sodium bouillons, including Featherweight and Lite-Line Low Sodium. These products contain only about 5 milligrams of sodium per serving. How can a flavorful bouillon be made without sodium? Most low-sodium bouillons are made with potassium chloride—the same ingredient found in salt substitutes—rather than sodium chloride (salt). However, if you are on a potassium-restricted diet, such products should be avoided.

Some of the most wholesome bouillon-type products available are the Vogue soup bases. Made mostly of powdered vegetables, soybeans, spices, and brewer's yeast, Vogue chicken, beef, onion, and vegetable bases contain about 300 milligrams of sodium per serving.

When shopping for your low-sodium bouillon, keep in mind that most products do contain monosodium glutamate or the related substances, hydrolyzed vegetable protein and hydrolyzed yeast extract. If these are ingredients that you're trying to avoid, read the label carefully before tossing the product into your shopping cart.

Dry Soup Mixes. The selection of low-fat, reduced-sodium dry soup offerings is not nearly as good as that of canned soups, but several brands are definitely worth stocking in your pantry. Fantastic Foods, Nile Spice, Dr. McDougall's Right Foods, and Health Valley make lines of dry soup mixes that are low in fat and contain less than 500 milligrams of sodium per serving. If 500 milligrams of sodium seems a bit high for a serving of soup, it is. But compared with the 1,000 or more milligrams of sodium in a traditional soup, 500 is pretty good—as long as you select lower-sodium foods to accompany your soup.

PASTAS AND SAUCES

Pasta makes a great quick meal—especially if you use a bottled sauce. And these days, there are several low-fat and fat-free brands from which to choose. As a rule, marinara (tomato based) sauces are much lower in fat than creamy white sauces. Ragu Light, Healthy Choice, and Muir Glen each feature an entire line of fat-free tomato pasta sauces that have only about 50 calories per half-cup serving. Compare this with brands made with oil, which can contain 6 or more grams of fat and 120 calories for the same-size serving, and your savings are clear. If you want a meat sauce, it is best to start with a fat-free marinara sauce. Then add your own 95-percent lean ground beef or turkey Italian sausage.

What about sodium? Many bottled marinara sauces—including the fat-free brands—contain close to 400 milligrams per half-cup serving, which is a sizable amount considering the suggested daily limit of 2,400 milligrams. However, several brands of low- and no-fat pasta sauces contain only 200 to 300 milligrams of sodium per serving. Among these are Millina's Finest Fat Free, Garden Valley Naturals Fat Free, and Mama Rizzo's Low Fat. For a no-salt-added low-fat sauce, try Eden Organic No Salt Added pasta sauce, or Enrico's All Natural No Salt Added sauces.

On those days when you have slightly more time—and a few minutes is all you'll need—it's easy to make a sauce that's practically sodium- and fat-free. Start with canned unsalted tomatoes like Eden No Salt Added tomatoes, Hunt's No Salt Added tomatoes, Del Monte No Salt Added stewed tomatoes, or Cento crushed tomatoes. Progresso Recipe Ready crushed tomatoes with added purée contains about half the sodium of most other brands, giving you a good start on a reduced-sodium sauce. Then add your own seasonings for a truly homemade taste. You can even afford to add some nonfat cheese or turkey Italian sausage and still remain well within your sodium budget.

As for the pasta itself, except for egg pastas, most are practically fat- and sodium-free. Keep in mind, though, that pastas are usually made from refined durum wheat flour, which, like other refined flours, lacks many of the nutrients found in whole grains.

A better choice is a whole wheat pasta. Some manufacturers, including De Bole's, Eden Foods, Hodgson Mill, Westbrae Natural, and Pritikin, offer some delicious whole wheat pastas. Now widely available, these pastas will add extra fiber and nutrients to your meal. What about Jerusalem artichoke pastas? A combination of durum wheat flour and Jerusalem artichoke flour, these products have a pleasant, slightly sweet flavor and smooth texture. Unless these pastas are made with whole grain durum wheat, however, they are no more nutritious than other refined pastas. For a nutritious artichoke-based pasta, look for De Bole's whole grain and Jerusalem artichoke products.

If you're looking for a change of pace, you may wish to try spinach or other vegetable pastas. Most brands do start out with refined durum wheat flour, but whole wheat vegetable pastas are also available. Are vegetable pastas more nutritious than plain pastas? It depends on the amount of vegetables added to the dough. Some brands of vegetable pastas do contain a significant amount of vitamin A from the added vegetables, but check the Nutrition Facts label to be sure.

If egg noodles are your pleasure, you will be happy to know that products like Mueller's Yolk Free noodles and No Yolks noodles contain the cholesterol-free egg whites only, making them great additions to a healthful meal.

MAYONNAISE, SALAD DRESSINGS, AND CONDIMENTS

Ingredients like mayonnaise, salad dressings, ketchup and mustard, and other condiments play a multitude of culinary roles, from dressing and binding salad ingredients, to moistening sandwich fillings, to adding zip to vegetable casseroles. And these days, there are just as many low-fat and no-fat options as there are oily, fatty ones. Let's take a look at some of the many products that can help you fight fat as you boost flavor.

Mayonnaise. Nonfat and reduced-fat mayonnaise are highly recommended over regular mayonnaise, which provides 10 grams of fat per tablespoon. How can mayonnaise be made without all that oil? Manufacturers use more water and vegetable thickeners to create creamy spreads that can replace the full-fat versions in all of your favorite recipes. Some widely available nonfat brands are Kraft Free, Miracle Whip Free, Smart Beat, and Weight Watchers Fat Free. In the low-fat category, you will find Hellmann's (Best Foods) Low Fat, with only 1 gram of fat per tablespoon, and Weight Watchers Light, with 2 grams of fat. A variety of reduced-fat brands are also available, with half to two thirds less fat and calories than regular mayonnaise. Look for brands like Hellmann's Light, Kraft Light, Miracle Whip Light, and Blue Plate Light.

Salad Dressings. Now made in a wide variety of flavors, fat-free dressings contain either no oil or so little oil that they have less than 0.5 gram of fat per 2-tablespoon serving. Compare the no- and low-fat products to their full-fat counterparts, which provide 12 to 18 grams of fat per 2-tablespoon serving, and your savings are clear. Use these dressings instead of oil-based brands to dress your favorite salads or as a delicious basting sauce for grilled foods. Look for nonfat brands like Good Seasons Fat Free, Hidden Valley Ranch Fat Free, Knott's Berry Farm Low Fat, Kraft Free, Marie's Fat Free, Pritikin, Marzetti's Fat Free, Seven Seas Free, Walden Farms Fat Free, and Wishbone Fat Free. Beware, though—many fat-free dressings are quite high in sodium, so compare brands and flavors, and choose those that are on the lower end of the sodium range. Another option is to dress your salads only with flavored vinegars. Try raspberry, rice, balsamic, herb, and red wine vinegars. And keep in mind that most vinegars are salt-free as well as fat-free.

Condiments. Condiments like mustard, ketchup, barbecue sauce, horseradish, soy sauce, Worcestershire sauce, and pepper sauce can really perk up an otherwise-bland dish. And, generally speaking, these ingredients are fat-free. The bad news is that many are quite high in sodium. In some cases, you will be able to find a lower-sodium version of your sauce. For instance, no-salt-added ketchups include Del Monte No Salt Added and Hunt's No Salt Added, while reduced-sodium products include Healthy Choice and Heinz Light Harvest. Reduced-sodium soy sauces include Kikkoman Lite, La Choy Lite, and Eden Reduced Sodium. When such alternatives are not available, limit the sodium content of your dish by avoiding the use of other salty ingredients.

JAMS, JELLIES, AND PRESERVES

Jams, jellies, and preserves have always been fat-free, and are good alternatives to butter and margarine for spreading on bread. What about calories? With just 16 calories per teaspoon, these products compare favorably to butter and margarine, which provide 45 calories per teaspoon. Reduced-sugar jams and jellies are also available, with half the calories of their full-sugar counterparts. Apple butter is another good choice for spreading on bread. And contrary to what the name implies, apple butter is fat-free.

How do all-fruit spreads stack up? The amount of calories and sugar in these products is generally not much different from that in sugar-sweetened spreads. The difference is that the sugar in all-fruit spreads comes from fruit and fruit juices instead of corn syrup or other refined sugars. Unfortunately, many brands of all-fruit spreads use highly refined, processed juices to sweeten their products, so nutritionally speaking, they are not much different from their sugar-sweetened counterparts. And you have no way of knowing just how refined the fruit juice sweetener is by looking at the label.

BAKING MIXES

Of all the Nutrition Facts labels, the labels on boxes of cake, brownie, cookie, muffin, and quick bread mixes are the most confusing and misleading. The reason? Calories are provided both for the mix alone and for the mix prepared according to package directions.

People often look only at the information for the mix, and disregard the Nutrition Facts for the prepared product—which includes the oil and eggs you add during mixing. Even worse, total fat grams are given only for the mix alone—not for the prepared product. For the prepared product, fat is expressed as a percentage of the Daily Value, a recommended daily amount based on a diet of 2,000 calories. This means that you can't readily see the dramatic rise in fat grams that occurs when the dry mix is combined with the necessary oil and eggs. Just how much fat gets added to your mix? Most cake mixes contain 2.5 to 5 grams of fat per serving in the mix alone. One third cup of oil and 3 eggs add another 7 grams of fat per serving—and that's before you ice or frost the cake.

But sometimes you can have your made-from-mix cake, muffins, brownies, and cookies, and eat them too. Lower-fat mixes for all of these products are available. Pillsbury Lovin' Lite brownie mixes; Betty Crocker Sweet Rewards reduced-fat and fat-free cake, brownie, and muffin mixes; SnackWell's low-fat and reduced-fat brownie and cake mixes; Krusteaz low-fat cookie and fat-free muffin mixes; and Krusteaz fat-free brownie mix are some examples. Products made from these mixes have just a fraction of the fat of those made from regular mixes.

However, you can just as easily take your favorite baking mix and make it lower in fat by replacing the oil or butter using the guidelines on page 95. Regular mixes prepared with fat substitutes will often have as little or even less fat than products made with light mixes. Bear in mind that even if you use a light mix or prepare a regular mix with fat substitutes, most of these products are high in sugar, refined flour, artificial ingredients, and calories. So while the finished product may be low in fat or even fat-free, it should have only a limited place in your diet. The exceptions to this rule are products made with whole grain mixes, like those by Arrowhead Mills. These mixes contain only whole grains, are low in sugar, and are free of artificial flavors, artificial colors, and other additives.

GRAINS AND FLOURS

Just because a food is fat-free does not mean it is good for you. Fat-free products made from refined white flour and refined grains are practically devoid of fiber, and contain few nutrients compared with their whole grain counterparts. In addition, fiber-rich foods are much more filling and satisfying than are refined products. Eating enough fiber is truly one of the secrets of low-fat living, as a diet of fat-free and low-fat refined foods is sure to leave you hungry. Fortunately, once accustomed to the heartier taste and texture of whole grains, most people prefer them over refined grains, which are bland and tasteless in comparison.

If you have never used whole grain flours before, a word should be said about storing these products. Since whole grain flours contain a very small amount of oil, they can more quickly become rancid than can their refined counterparts. For this reason, be sure to store them in the refrigerator or freezer.

Not sure how to substitute whole grain flours for the refined flours in your favorite recipes? The guidelines in Chapter 5 will make it easy for you to successfully replace part or all of the refined flour with one of the healthy whole grain products discussed below.

Barley. This grain has a light, nutty flavor, making it a great substitute for rice in pilafs, soups, casseroles, and other dishes. Hulled barley, like brown rice, cooks in about 50 minutes. Quick-cooking barley is also widely available. With all the fiber of hulled barley, this product, available from both Mother's and Quaker, cooks in about 12 minutes. **Barley flour** is also available in health foods stores and some grocery stores. This mildly sweet flour is perfect for cakes, muffins, and other baked goods, and can replace up to a third of the wheat flour in these products.

Brown Rice. Brown rice is whole-kernel rice, meaning that all nutrients are intact. With a slightly chewy texture and a pleasant nutty flavor, brown rice makes excellent pilafs and stuffings. Brown rice does take twice as long as white rice to cook. But if you place the rice in the cooking water and refrigerate it overnight, or for at least 8 hours, the grain will cook in just 20 to 25 minutes. Several brands of quick-cooking brown rice—including Arrowhead Mills, Minute Brand, and Uncle Ben's—are also widely available. These brands can be made in 10 to 12 minutes. **Brown rice flour** is also available in many grocery stores and makes a nutritious addition to waffles, cookies, and other baked goods, where it adds a pleasant crunchy texture.

Buckwheat. Buckwheat is technically not a grain, but the edible fruit seed of a plant that is closely related to rhubarb. Roasted buckwheat kernels, commonly known as **kasha,** are delicious in pilafs and hot breakfast cereals. **Buckwheat flour,** made from finely ground whole buckwheat kernels, is delicious in pancakes, waffles, breads, and muffins.

Cornmeal. This grain adds a sweet flavor, a lovely golden color, and a crunchy texture to baked goods. Select whole grain (unbolted) cornmeal for the most nutrition. Your next best choice is bolted cornmeal, which is nearly whole grain. By contrast, degermed cornmeal is refined. Look for brands like Arrowhead Mills and Hodgson Mill in your local grocery and health foods stores.

Oats. Loaded with cholesterol-lowering soluble fiber, oats aren't just for breakfast. Use this healthful product to add a chewy texture and sweet flavor to muffins, quick breads, pancakes, cookies, and crumb toppings.

Another fiber-rich product to look for is **oat bran.** Made of the outer part of the oat kernel, oat bran has a sweet, mild flavor and is a concentrated source of cholesterol-lowering soluble fiber. Great as a hot and hearty breakfast cereal, oat bran can also replace part of the flour in your low-fat baked goods, where it helps to retain moisture. Look for oat bran in the hot cereal section of your grocery store alongside the rolled oats. The softer, more finely ground products, like Quaker and Mother's, can be substituted for up to a third of the flour in baked goods. Coarsely ground oat brans, like Hodgson Mill, add a pleasantly chewy texture to muffins and cookies. When using a coarsely ground product, soak it in some of the recipe's liquid for about 15 minutes before adding it to the recipe.

Still another oat product to stock up on is **oat flour.** This mildly sweet flour is perfect for cakes, muffins, and other baked goods. Like oat bran, oat flour retains moisture in baked goods, reducing the need for fat. To add extra fiber and nutrients, substitute oat flour for up to a third of the refined wheat flour in your own recipes. Look for Arrowhead Mills oat flour in grocery and health foods stores, or make your own oat flour by grinding quick-cooking rolled oats in a blender.

Unbleached Flour. This is refined white flour that has not been subjected to a bleaching process. Unbleached white flour lacks significant amounts of nutrients compared with whole wheat flour, but does contain more vitamin E than bleached flour. Arrowhead Mills, Gold Medal, Hodgson Mill, and Pillsbury's Best all make unbleached flour.

White Whole Wheat Flour. This is an excellent whole grain flour for all your baking needs. Made from hard white wheat instead of the hard red wheat used to make regular whole wheat flour, white wheat flour contains all the fiber and nutrients of regular whole wheat flour, but is sweeter and lighter tasting than its red wheat counterpart. King Arthur white whole wheat flour is available in many grocery stores.

Whole Grain Wheat. Available in many forms, this grain is perhaps easiest to use in the form of bulgur wheat. Cracked wheat that is precooked and dried, bulgur wheat can be prepared in a matter of minutes and can replace rice in any recipe. Look for it in grocery and health foods stores.

Whole Wheat Flour. Made of ground whole grain wheat kernels, whole wheat flour includes the grain's nutrient-rich bran and germ. Nutritionally speaking, whole wheat flour is far superior to refined flour. Sadly, many people grew up eating refined baked goods and find whole grain products too heavy for their taste. A good way to learn to enjoy whole grain flours is to use part whole wheat and part unbleached flour in recipes, and gradually increase the amount of whole wheat used over time. Most grocery stores stock Gold Medal, Pillsbury's Best, Hodgson Mill, Arrowhead Mills, or Heckers whole wheat flour. If you find these brands too heavy for your taste, try either whole wheat pastry flour or white whole wheat flour.

Whole Wheat Pastry Flour. When muffin, quick bread, cake, pastry, pancake, pie crust, and cookie recipes call for whole wheat flour, whole wheat pastry flour is the best choice. The reason? Made from a finely ground, soft (low-protein) wheat, whole wheat pastry flour produces lighter, softer-textured baked goods than regular whole wheat flour does. Look for Arrowhead Mills whole wheat pastry flour in health foods stores and many grocery stores. Keep in mind, though, that whole wheat pastry flour is not suitable for most yeast breads. Regular whole wheat and white whole wheat flours, which are higher in gluten, will allow your yeast breads to rise better.

THE FREEZER CASE

The freezer case offers a good selection of time-saving products, from vegetables to entrées, pizzas, and desserts. Let's take a look at the best fat-saving products from this section of the grocery store.

Frozen Vegetables. Many busy people love the convenience of frozen vegetables. Your best bet when buying frozen vegetables is to choose the unsauced, unseasoned versions, and then add your own seasonings. By doing this, you will avoid unwanted salt and fat, and you will save money. These days, a number of interesting frozen vegetable combinations—such as stir-fry vegetables, Italian vegetable blend, and gumbo vegetables—are available to cook and eat as a side dish or to use in recipes.

Looking for low-fat frozen fries? Think big. The larger the cut, the less surface area there is to soak up fat. Large-cut fries like Ore Ida Potato Wedges With Skins have only 2.5 grams of fat per serving, rather than the 5 or 6 fat grams found in a serving of thinner-cut shoestring fries. Finally, to keep the fat count low, be sure to bake those fries in the oven instead of deep-frying them.

Frozen Dinners, Entrées, and Pizzas. Today's busy lifestyles make frozen dinners a popular alternative to cooking. In the past, most brands of frozen dinners and entrées contained too much fat, too much salt, or too much of both to be a regular part of a prudent diet. Fortunately, this no longer holds true. Manufacturers have responded to consumer demand, and healthier options that are low in both fat and salt are now widely available.

Healthy Choice was the first company to offer an entire line of low-fat dinners and entrées that were not loaded with sodium, and their popularity with consumers led to a revolution in the frozen food case. All Healthy Choice meals get well under 30 percent of their calories from fat and contain less than 600 milligrams of sodium. Brands like Tyson, Budget Gourmet Light and Healthy, Lean Cuisine, and Weight Watchers also offer many products that meet these same guidelines. How can you spot the best fat-fighting frozen dinners and entrées? Simply read the Nutrition Facts information. If your frozen meal contains less than 10 grams of fat and less than 600 milligrams of sodium, you should be able to stay within the bounds of your daily fat and sodium budgets.

One type of frozen entrée that is especially popular is the pizza. Happily, when made properly, pizza is not a junk food, but an excellent low-fat source of calcium, carbohydrates, and other nutrients. The freezer case of your local grocery store most likely has several brands of reduced-fat pizzas. Leading the low-fat pack are Stouffer's Lean Cuisine French Bread Pizza, Healthy Choice French Bread Pizza, Tombstone Light Vegetable Pizza, and Weight Watchers Deluxe Combo Pizza. These brands get from 16 to 26 percent of their calories from fat. As a basis of comparison, keep in mind that regular frozen pizzas—even vegetable pizzas—get close to half their calories from fat.

Many people complain that they still feel hungry after eating a frozen meal or entrée. If this is true of you, realize that an entire meal which supplies less than 300 calories won't stick with most people for more than a couple of hours—if, in fact, it satisfies them at all. Surprisingly, frozen meals tend to fall short in the vegetable department, with most providing less than a one-cup serving of this very important food group. For this reason, these dinners also often supply insufficient amounts of vitamins A and C, and dietary fiber. The solution? Add a salad—with nonfat dressing—or a piece of fruit to your meal. Unless your entrée is bread based, like pizza, also add a piece of whole grain bread. These additions will provide nutritional balance and keep you feeling full and satisfied until the next meal.

Frozen Desserts. Unlike cookies, cakes, and other sugary treats, frozen dairy desserts do provide some nutritional value. One cup of most brands of low- or no-fat frozen yogurt or ice cream supplies 20 to 30 percent of the Daily Value for calcium. And, of course, these brands save you an astounding amount of fat over full-fat premium products, which can contain about 40 grams per cup!

Look for brands with no more than 3 grams of fat per one-cup serving. Good choices include Ben & Jerry's no-fat frozen yogurt, Borden Fat Free ice cream, Breyers Fat Free ice cream and frozen yogurt, Colombo Nonfat frozen yogurt, Crowley Nonfat frozen yogurt, Dannon Light frozen yogurt, Haagen Daz Fat-Free frozen yogurt and Low-Fat frozen yogurt bars, Healthy Choice Premium Low Fat ice cream, Edy's Fat Free ice cream and frozen yogurt, Sealtest Free ice cream, and Stonyfield Farm Nonfat frozen yogurt. When perusing the frozen foods case, note that most ice cream packages list their serving size as a half cup, but most people eat a full cup.

Other frozen treats to look for include sherbets, sorbets, and ices, most of which have always been fat-free; Dole Fruit Juice and Fruit 'n' Juice bars; Welch's fruit juice bars; and fat-free fudgsicles.

PACKAGED SIDE DISHES

Many busy people love the convenience of boxed side dish mixes. Whether the dish is macaroni and cheese, potatoes au gratin, or rice pilaf, most of the ingredients are in the box, and with a minimum of effort, you can enjoy a tasty dish in just a few minutes.

The bad news is that while side dish mixes are convenient, most are highly processed, and therefore high in sodium and artificial ingredients. In fact, a half-cup serving of most mixes provides 500 to 700 milligrams of sodium. Most rice and pasta side dish mixes are made with white rice and refined pasta, so that they contain significantly less fiber, vitamins, and minerals than whole grain products. And if your family loves mashed potatoes made from potato flakes, or other dishes made with dehydrated potatoes, keep in mind that processing has robbed these potatoes of most of their vitamin C. To make matters worse, many side dish mixes also call for unhealthy amounts of fat to be added during preparation.

Fortunately, side-by-side with these high-sodium, highly processed products are some excellent packaged side dishes that are easy to make, low in fat, and just as delicious as their higher-sodium and -fat counterparts. Moreover, a number of regular side dish mixes can be made low-fat with a just a few ingredient substitutions.

Most grocery and health foods stores offer a number of healthful packaged side dishes. Arrowhead Mills, for instance, makes a variety of quick-cooking brown rice pilafs—products that provide lots of flavor and nutrition with far less sodium than most brands. Lundberg Farms, Near East, Fantastic Foods, and De Bole's also make a range of whole grain side dish mixes, from macaroni and cheese to brown rice and lentil pilafs.

When whipping up side dishes with *any* mix, it's easy to make a healthier dish by modifying the manufacturer's directions. In fact, many mixes, as packaged, contain very little fat. Most of the finished dish's fat is added during preparation. When preparing your favorite packaged mix, simply replace the full-fat products called for with their no- or low-fat counterparts. For instance, if the directions on a box of macaroni and cheese instruct you to add milk and margarine to the sauce packet, substitute skim milk and reduced-fat or nonfat margarine. Or use only the skim milk, and leave out the margarine entirely. If the resulting sauce seems a little dry, add a few more tablespoons of milk until the sauce has the desired consistency. You'll soon learn the best way to prepare the mix so that the dish is both healthy and tasty.

THE PRODUCE DEPARTMENT

This is one part of the supermarket where we should all spend more time. Why? To maximize your health, nothing is more important than eating at least five servings of fruits and vegetables each day. With a few exceptions, produce is fat-free. Moreover, all produce is cholesterol-free and rich in the fiber and nutrients that help ward off cancer, heart disease, and many other disorders.

Contrary to popular belief, produce is fast food—or, at least, it should be. The fact is that the less you do to fresh fruits and vegetables in the way of cooking, the more nutritious they are. Vegetables served raw in salads, steamed, or stir-fried only until crisp-tender are just what the doctor ordered. Prepared in these ways, produce requires very little time. And what could be a faster snack than a piece of fresh fruit eaten out of hand?

Although all produce provides fiber and nutrients for very few calories, some fruits and vegetables are especially rich in nutrients. Some of the best vegetable selections include those in the cabbage family, such as broccoli, bok choy, cabbage, cauliflower, kale, and greens. Carrots, sweet peppers, sweet potatoes, tomatoes, and winter squash are other nutrient-packed choices. Supernutritious fruits include oranges, mangoes, cantaloupes, kiwi, and strawberries. Try to eat these foods often.

Selecting Produce

Buy fresh, locally grown produce whenever possible. This will help insure that the produce you buy is more nutritious, and grown with fewer pesticides and chemicals. If local produce is not available, domestically grown produce is a better choice than imported produce. Why? Most other countries are allowed to use harmful pesticides and other chemicals that are banned in the United States. Of course, your best option, whenever possible, is to purchase organic produce, which is grown without chemical fertilizers and pesticides of any kind. It is also a very good idea to purchase fruits and vegetables in season. By doing this, you will be much more likely to get a juicy, flavorful, and nutritious product for the best value.

Is fresh always best? Yes—if the produce has been properly handled. Beware, though. If fresh produce was picked when underripe, mishandled during shipping, and then stored for several days before being sold, frozen vegetables are a better option. Frozen vegetables are picked close to their peak of ripeness and then quickly processed, allowing them to retain more nutrients than poorly handled fresh produce. Even canned vegetables may be more nutritious than some fresh vegetables.

As you walk through the produce section of your grocery store, you will often see people squeezing, thumping, shaking, and sniffing the merchandise, checking for ripeness and freshness. How can you choose the best produce? Look for vegetables and fruits that are plump and heavy for their size. This indicates that the produce is juicy, rather than dried out. Avoid any produce that looks shriveled or wilted, and therefore past its prime. Also avoid produce that is overly large, as this may indicate a stringy texture and bitter taste. Finally, check the item for fragrance. Fruit that has a sweet smell is at its peak of ripeness and flavor. Fruits such as strawberries and blueberries should be purchased when fully mature and ripe. Fruits such as bananas, pears, kiwi, cantaloupes, plums, peaches, and nectarines may be purchased slightly underripe and allowed to finish ripening at room temperature at home. Place the produce in a closed paper bag to hasten the process. Avoid fruits that are very firm or hard and have a greenish color, as these were probably picked when immature and will never ripen properly.

Avoiding the Fat Traps

Although you can make most of your purchases in the produce department without fear of fat, there are a few exceptions. Coconut and avocados are two fruits that are loaded with fat.

In the case of coconut, the fat is of the highly saturated, artery-clogging kind. This is not to say that you should entirely eliminate coconut from your diet. Rather, use it sparingly. Try adding some coconut-flavored extract to cakes, cookies, muffins, and other baked goods to reduce the need for flaked or shredded coconut. A few tablespoons of coconut may then be all that is needed.

As for avocados, their fat is mostly monounsaturated, which has no harmful health effects other than being high in calories, like all fats. Moreover, these velvety fruits are rich in vitamin E, potassium, folate, vitamin B_6, and other nutrients. So if you like avocados, by all means, work them into your fat budget. Even with 11.5 grams of fat and 121 calories per half cup, the avocado is certainly a better fat choice than a tablespoon of butter, margarine, or oil, which provides about the same amount of fat and calories.

Nuts are another food that can lure you into the fat trap. These tasty morsels add crunch and flavor to a variety of dishes. Unfortunately, they also add fat and calories—about 80 grams of fat and 800 calories per cup. But take heart. Like avocados, nuts are high in monounsaturated fats, and so do not promote heart disease. In fact, some studies show that people who eat nuts on a regular basis actually *lower* their risk of heart disease. The reason for this may be that the fat in nuts—unlike the fat in refined oils—still contains all of its vitamin E and other essential nutrients. So if you like nuts, feel free to spend some of your fat budget on them. Instead of eating them by the handful, though, sprinkle a few over salads, add some to casseroles, or stir 3 or 4 tablespoons into muffin, quick bread, and cake batters.

To get the most out of nuts, try toasting them. Toasting intensifies the flavor of nuts so much that you can often halve the amount used. (For directions on toasting nuts, see page 80.) This will help you add flavor and a nutritious crunch to your dishes *without* blowing your fat budget.

Preparing Produce

Once you've brought your produce home, you'll want to prepare it in a way that maximizes taste and nutrition. If your produce is not organic, be sure to peel or thoroughly wash it before using. If any of your produce is waxed—and many apples, cucumbers, eggplants, and other fruits and vegetables are—peeling will be your best bet, as waxes cannot be washed away. For maximum freshness and nutritional value, wash and cut your vegetables just before cooking. Washing and cutting hours before use can destroy nutrients.

Finally, to preserve vitamins and minerals, eat vegetables raw, or cook them in a steamer or microwave oven just until crisp-tender. Vegetables that are cooked just until done retain not only their nutrients, but also their appealing color and fresh taste.

SWEET TREATS

The past few years have brought a multitude of fat-free and low-fat ways to satisfy a sweet tooth. Cookies, brownies, cakes, pies, and pastries are all now being made with little or no fat. Unfortunately, as many weight-conscious people have discovered, many of these products, while lower in fat, fall short of what you might wish them to be both nutritionally and as a means of controlling weight. A glance at the Nutrition Facts label on many no- and low-fat baked goods and frozen desserts reveals that when fat is removed, sugar is often added. The result? The fat content of the product is lower, but, very often, the calorie count has not been greatly changed.

Are reduced-fat sweets an improvement over their high-fat counterparts? Yes, but nutritional powerhouses they are not. In fact, most of these products are made from nutrient-poor refined grains and with an abundance of sugar and artificial ingredients. For this reason, when choosing any sweets, let not only your fat budget, but also your sugar budget (about 40 to 50 grams a day) and calorie budget be your guide. With these guidelines in mind, let's take a look at some of the no- and low-fat products that can make your snack and dessert times a little bit sweeter. (To learn about frozen desserts, see page 64.)

Cookies and Brownies. An amazing array of fat-free and low-fat cookies are now available at your local grocery store. Your best bets are cookies that are lower on both the sugar end and the fat end. Examples are most brands of low-fat graham crackers, low-fat vanilla or chocolate wafers, animal crackers, and low-fat gingersnaps. Frookie Fat Free, Health Valley, Jammers, Nabisco Newtons, SnackWell's cinnamon grahams, SnackWell's oatmeal raisin, and Sunshine Golden Fruit biscuits are other good choices. Besides being fat-free, Health Valley and Jammers are made with whole grain flours.

As for fat-free and low-fat brownies, most brands deliver 4 to 5 teaspoons of sugar (16 to 20 grams) apiece. Still, the reduced-fat versions are a better option than those made with fat. Famous Amos, Greenfield, Pepperidge Farm, Jammers, SnackWell's, and many other companies offer these nonfat and low-fat treats.

Granola Bars. In years past, granola bars were little more than candy bars in disguise, with unhealthy amounts of fat and sugar wrapped around otherwise healthful oats and other grains. These days, many brands of granola bars have really lightened up, making them a far better snack choice than most cookies. Select brands like Fibar Low Fat, Health Valley, Kellogg's Low Fat, Kudos Low Fat, Quaker Low Fat, and Nature Valley Low Fat. But don't think you're filling up with fiber when you eat a granola bar. With the exception of Health Valley and Fibar granola bars, most contain only 1 gram of fiber. Still, these products do contain more whole grains than most cookies, and tend to be lower in sugar, too.

Cakes, Pies, and Pastries. In this category, Entenmann's has developed an extensive line of fat-free and low-fat cakes, Danish pastries, pies, and other goodies. Hostess also offers some fat-free and low-fat baked goods. Like all sweets, though, these should be considered an occasional indulgence.

Perhaps the best cake choice of all has been around for years—angel food cake. This sweet treat has always been fat-free. Topped with fresh fruit, it makes a light, elegant, and comparatively low-sugar dessert.

THE SNACK AISLE

Until recently, dedicated fat-fighters had few options in the snack aisle. But all that has changed. These days, there are plenty of excellent low- and no-fat chips, pretzels, and other fun foods that take the guilt out of snacking while leaving in the flavor and crunch. Let's take a look at some of the many products that await you at your local grocery store.

Crackers. Although plenty of fat-free and low-fat options abound in the cracker aisle, your best bets are crackers that are both low in fat and high in whole grains. Brands like Ak-Mak, Finn Crisp, Health Valley, Hol Grain, Kavli, Ry-Krisp, Ryvita, Wasa, and Manischewitz Whole Wheat Matzos are among the most healthful choices. Other good options are rice and popcorn cakes, most of which are made with whole grains and little or no added fat. Reduced-Fat Triscuits and Reduced-Fat Wheat Thins also provide some fiber, but with a little more fat.

Next in line are crackers that are fat-free or low in fat, but contain mostly refined white flour or refined grains. These include Mr. Phipps Fat-Free Pretzel Chips, Barbara's Low-Fat, Hain Low-Fat, Jacobsen's Snack Toast, the SnackWell's line of crackers, Stoned Wheat Thins, fat-free saltines, and melba toast.

As a hearty and nutritious alternative to crackers and rice cakes, accompany your favorite dips and spreads with wedges of whole grain pita bread, slices of firm whole wheat or rye bread, or slices of whole grain bagels.

Chips. To the delight of chip lovers everywhere, several brands of low-fat and fat-free potato chips are now widely available. These crispy chips—which are baked, not fried—make a tasty snack. Look for brands like Baked Lay's, Childer's Fat Free, Fit Foods Fat Free, Louise's Fat Free and Low-Fat, and many others. If tortilla chips are more to your liking, try a brand like Baked Tostitos, Guiltless Gourmet, Louise's, or Smart Temptations. In each case, you will save about 10 grams of fat and 60 calories per ounce of chips. And most brands of fat-free chips have surprisingly little sodium— about 100 to 200 milligrams per 1-ounce serving. Unsalted brands are also available.

Popcorn. It's hard to beat air-popped popcorn as a snack food. For buttery flavor, spray your air-popped treat with a little Weight Watchers Butter Spray or I Can't Believe It's Not Butter! spray. In the microwave popcorn department, look for brands like Orville Redenbacher's Smart Pop, Weight Watchers Smart Snackers Microwave Popcorn, or Betty Crocker Pop Secret by Request.

Pretzels. While these crunchy treats have always been low in fat, most pretzels are little more than refined white flour and salt. And with up to 600 milligrams of sodium per 1-ounce serving, your average pretzel is not the most nutritious snack-food choice.

Fortunately, some unsalted and reduced-salt brands are available, including Bachman unsalted and Quinlan unsalted. And some pretzels do contain whole grain flour. One good choice is Wege Honey Wheat pretzels. Made with part whole wheat flour and coated with sesame seeds, these pretzels make a satisfying snack that is low in both fat and salt. Yet another excellent product is Barbara's Organic Whole Wheat Pretzels.

Salsa. Once you have selected a bag of low-fat chips or a box of low-fat crackers, you may be faced with a real challenge—finding a healthy dip in a sea of high-fat, high-sodium products. Try salsa, which has always been fat-free. Compare brands, though, and choose those with the lowest sodium counts. Green Mountain Gringo, Louise's, and Guiltless Gourmet salsas tend to be lower in sodium than most other brands. Enrico's and Millina's Finest both offer salsas made with no added salt. And don't forget that for a creamy guilt-free treat, you can easily prepare your favorite chip dip using nonfat sour cream.

Now that you know about all the excellent no- and low-fat products that are available, you are ready to begin creating healthful low-fat dishes. In the next chapter, you'll learn the simple cooking techniques that will allow you to use these products with delicious results each and every time you cook.

5. Secrets of Cooking Fat-Free

F or many years, cooking healthfully meant limited food choices and—all too often—bland and boring results. Fortunately, those days are over. Now, fat-free foods can be varied and delicious, and cooking fat-free can be a rewarding adventure.

The biggest boon to the fat-free cook was the development of many excellent fat-saving products. From sour cream and cheese to bacon and sausage, there is now a low- or no-fat alternative to just about any ingredient you want to use. As a result, a variety of previously forbidden dishes, like crispy fried chicken and tantalizing spaghetti carbonara, can now be made fat-free and delicious.

But there's more to fat-free cooking than simply substituting low-fat ingredients for their high-fat counterparts. The cooking characteristics of a number of the new low- and no-fat ingredients are different from those of the ingredients they are replacing, so that slight recipe modifications are sometimes needed to insure success. Moreover, it is useful to know about the many innovative cooking techniques—like braising, blackening, and baking in parchment paper—that can help you slash the fat and enhance the flavor of a wide variety of foods.

This chapter presents the tricks of the trade that will help you successfully use lower-fat products in your favorite recipes. You will also discover how fat-free cooking techniques and the skillful use of seasonings can bring out the best in all your foods. You will even learn how to make your favorite baked goods with far less fat. Believe it or not, even rich and creamy cheesecakes can be part of a healthy diet—once you know the secrets of cooking fat-free.

SUBSTITUTIONS THAT SLASH FAT AND CALORIES

A handful of ingredients—like butter, margarine, oil, mayonnaise, cheese, and cream—add the majority of fat to most dishes. Fortunately, there are plenty of healthful substitutes that can reduce calories and fat without sacrificing flavor. This section shares the techniques that will allow you to successfully eliminate the most common high-fat ingredients from your favorite dishes.

Cooking With Low- and Nonfat Cheeses

Cheese is one of those foods that few people are willing to give up. Fortunately, there's no need to anymore. Whether you like your cheese melted atop a pizza or whipped into a creamy cheesecake, a wide range of nonfat and low-fat products is now available, making it possible for even the most discriminating fat-fighters to have their cheese and eat it, too.

Cooking With Firm and Hard Cheeses

While low- and no-fat firm and hard cheeses are a great addition to the fat-free kitchen, using these products successfully in cooked dishes does require a little know-how. Here are some tips for working with these great fat-saving foods.

☐ When using nonfat cheeses to make a cheese sauce, a cheese soup, or other dishes in which you want the cheese to melt smoothly, use a finely shredded brand. Often referred to on the package label as "fancy" shredded cheese, finely shredded nonfat cheeses melt better than coarsely shredded brands—although they still may not melt completely. Another option is to use a process nonfat cheese. Process cheeses are specially made to melt, so they will work in any sauce recipe. Most process cheeses tend to be quite high in sodium, but you can avoid a sodium overload when using these cheeses by leaving out the salt and avoiding the use of other high-sodium ingredients in your recipe. What about reduced-fat cheeses? Most brands melt nicely, and can be substituted for full-fat brands in any sauce recipe, with very little difference in taste or texture.

Here's a tip for perking up low-fat and nonfat cheese sauces. Add a little dry mustard to the sauce. This pungent spice enhances the flavor of many cheeses, especially Cheddar cheese. How much should you use? Start with $1/4$ teaspoon of dry mustard per cup of milk, and add more if desired. When making Swiss or Parmesan cheese sauces, try adding a pinch of ground nutmeg to bring out the flavor.

☐ When topping a casserole with nonfat cheese, sprinkle the cheese on top and bake the casserole covered, removing the cover during the last 10 minutes of baking. Or add the cheese only during the last 5 to 10 minutes of baking. This will prevent the cheese from becoming dry and rubbery. Of course, as explained above, low-fat cheeses melt more smoothly and completely than their nonfat counterparts, so these modifications are usually not necessary when using a low-fat product.

☐ Top your favorite pizza with either nonfat or low-fat cheese. Keep in mind, though, that reduced-fat brands, like Sargento Light Shredded Mozzarella, will have more "stretch" than nonfat brands. You can also mix equal parts of shredded nonfat mozzarella and shredded reduced-fat provolone. This will give you the texture you love, but with about two thirds less fat than you'd get with a full-fat cheese.

☐ When topping salads, tacos, or a bowl of chili or black bean soup, enjoy great results with *any* of the nonfat or low-fat shredded brands. Only your waistline will know the difference between these cheeses and a full-fat product!

Cooking With Parmesan Cheese

A favorite pasta topping, this popular cheese is so flavorful that a little bit goes a long way. One tablespoon of full-fat Parmesan contains just under 2 grams of fat, so used in moderate amounts, even the regular cheese can have a place in your low-fat diet. But by using nonfat Parmesan in recipes that call for large amounts of this cheese, you will greatly reduce the fat content of the finished dish.

☐ Substitute a nonfat or reduced-fat brand of Parmesan for the full-fat version in recipes like fettuccine Alfredo, lasagna, and other pasta dishes. Either type will work well.

☐ Use nonfat Parmesan—which contains added starches—to help thicken cream soups and sauces. Add the Parmesan toward the end of the cooking time, stirring in about 1 tablespoon of cheese per cup of liquid. Let the soup or sauce simmer for a minute or 2 to thicken. Then, if desired, add a bit more cheese for a thicker consistency. Be sure to reduce or eliminate the salt in the recipe, as Parmesan already contains salt.

☐ When topping casseroles with nonfat Parmesan, sprinkle the cheese on top and bake the casserole covered, removing the cover during the last 10 minutes of baking. This will prevent the top from becoming dry. Or top your casserole with regular Parmesan. Three tablespoons sprinkled over a casserole that serves six people will add only 1 gram of fat per serving.

☐ To add extra cheese flavor to your homemade low-fat pizzas, sprinkle a tablespoon or two of nonfat Parmesan over the tomato sauce layer of the pizza. Then add the mozzarella and any other toppings of your choice.

Cooking With Reduced- and Nonfat Cream Cheese

Nonfat cream cheese, light cream cheese, and Neufchâtel can all replace their full-fat counterparts in dips and spreads, casseroles, and cheesecakes. Use the following guidelines to get the best results.

☐ When using nonfat cream cheese in recipes, be sure to use the block-style product rather than the tub-style, which is meant for spreading. Since the block cream cheese contains less water, it will perform better in your low-fat recipes.

☐ Since even the block-style nonfat cream cheese contains more water than full-fat cream cheese, you may have to adjust your recipes for the best results. For instance, when using nonfat cream cheese in cheesecakes, you may find that the texture of the cake is softer—more pudding-like—than that of traditional cheesecake. If so, try adding a tablespoon of flour to the batter for each cup of nonfat cream cheese used. This should produce a firm, nicely textured cake that is remarkably low in calories and fat.

☐ If you've ever tried to defat a cream cheese frosting recipe by substituting fat-free cream cheese for the full-fat product, you probably ended up with a runny, watery mess. This is because when more than a couple of tablespoons of sugar is added to fat-free cream cheese, the cheese's water is released, resulting in a runny glaze. The solution? Make the frosting with Neufchâtel, a reduced-fat cheese. Or beat in a tablespoon or two of instant vanilla pudding mix. This will thicken the mixture to the desired consistency.

☐ Another excellent substitute for cream cheese is yogurt cheese. This product can easily be made at home by following the simple directions presented in the inset "Making Yogurt Cheese," found below.

☐ Try using soft curd farmer cheese to replace the cream cheese in dips, spreads, cheesecakes, creamy fillings, and many other recipes. Just be sure to read the package label before you make your purchase, as some brands are made with whole milk.

Cooking With Reduced- and Nonfat Ricotta Cheese

Many brands of nonfat ricotta cheese are available to save fat and calories in your favorite dishes. Here are some ways to use this nutritious product.

☐ Substitute nonfat ricotta for the whole milk variety in lasagna, manicotti, white pizza, and other dishes. Nonfat cottage cheese can also replace ricotta in dishes like lasagna and manicotti.

☐ When using nonfat ricotta in a creamy mixture that also contains sugar—in cake fillings, for instance—be careful not to add more than a couple of tablespoons of sugar per cup of ricotta. Because nonfat ricotta has a high water content, more than a little sugar can cause the mixture to become runny.

☐ When making tiramisu and similar desserts, substitute puréed nonfat ricotta cheese for high-fat mascarpone cheese. Or purée equal parts of nonfat ricotta and nonfat or light cream cheese.

Making Yogurt Cheese

Yogurt cheese—a great substitute for cream cheese—is a wonderfully versatile food that can be used in dips and spreads, or even baked in cheesecakes by using it to replace the usual cream cheese.

When using yogurt cheese in your recipes, for best results, avoid using a blender or food processor for mixing, as this can cause the cheese to thin. Instead, gently mix this ingredient into dips, spreads, and other mixtures with a spoon or a wire whisk. When making cheesecakes, substitute yogurt cheese for cream cheese on a cup-for-cup basis, adding 1 tablespoon of flour for each cup of yogurt cheese used. This will insure a firm-textured yet creamy cake.

To make yogurt cheese, start with any brand of fat-free or low-fat plain or flavored yogurt that does not contain gelatin. Simply place the yogurt in a funnel lined with cheesecloth or a coffee filter, and let it drain into a jar in the refrigerator for 8 hours or overnight. Special funnels designed just for making yogurt cheese are also available in cooking shops. When the yogurt is reduced by half, it is ready to use. The whey that collects in the jar may be used in bread and muffin recipes, in place of the listed liquid.

☐ Use nonfat ricotta cheese, as is or lightly sweetened, as a creamy filling for blintzes.

☐ Try substituting nonfat ricotta for part of the cream cheese in cheesecakes. To maintain a firm texture, add a tablespoon of flour for each cup of nonfat ricotta used.

☐ Use puréed nonfat ricotta to add delightful creaminess to mousses, gelatin molds, and other uncooked dishes.

Cooking With Reduced-Fat and Nonfat Margarine and Butter

With up to 11 less grams of fat per tablespoon compared with their full-fat counterparts, low- and no-fat margarine and butter are well worth using both at the table and in your cooking. Here are some ideas for using these fat-fighting ingredients in your favorite dishes.

☐ For the majority of your cooking and spreading needs, switch to a reduced-fat brand of butter or margarine that contains 3 to 6 grams of fat per tablespoon. Although these products are not well-suited for sautéing, they can be tossed with steamed vegetables, and can deliciously replace regular butter and margarine in pasta and rice dishes, sauces, casseroles, and many other dishes. Reduced-fat butter and margarine can also be used to coat the outside of your bread when making grilled cheese sandwiches.

☐ Use nonfat margarines, which are now available for spreading on breads and other foods, in dishes like mashed potatoes. These products also melt well enough to be tossed with hot pasta and rice, or to be used in some casseroles and other dishes. Again, nonfat margarine is not recommended for sautéing.

☐ In side dish mixes—like macaroni and cheese—whose directions require the addition of butter or margarine, try eliminating the butter or margarine by substituting an equal amount of skim milk or nonfat sour cream. Or use nonfat margarine.

☐ Use butter-flavored sprinkles like Molly McButter and Butter Buds to add buttery flavor to recipes. A couple of teaspoons stirred into sauces, casseroles, rice, steamed vegetables, and other dishes add the taste of butter without the fat. Butter Buds also comes in packets that you mix with water to make a pourable butter substitute that works nicely in sauces and many other dishes. Butter Buds liquid cannot be used for sautéing, however.

☐ Replace the butter or margarine in stuffings with broth or Butter Buds liquid. Start by adding half as much broth or Butter Buds as the amount of margarine called for. Then mix up the stuffing—it should be moist and hold together nicely. Add more fat substitute if needed.

☐ For ideas on reducing and eliminating butter and margarine in your baked goods, see the baking tips on pages 96 to 101.

Cooking With Cream Substitutes

With 821 calories and 88 grams per cup, cream can blow your fat budget in a hurry. But don't fear; several nonfat products can beautifully replace this high-fat ingredient. As a bonus, these healthful substitutes will add some calcium and other nutrients to your dish.

☐ Substitute evaporated skimmed milk on a one-for-one basis for the cream in quiches, sauces, cream soups, custards, puddings, and many other dishes. A wonderful cooking aid, this product adds creamy richness but no fat.

☐ For another excellent cream substitute, mix $^1/_3$ cup of nonfat dry milk powder with 1 cup of skim milk. Use this mixture as you would evaporated skimmed milk to replace the cream in any recipe. Or stir a few tablespoons of nonfat dry milk powder into cream soups, sauces, custards, and puddings to add creamy richness while boosting nutritional value. For best results, always buy *instant* nonfat dry milk powder, as this product will not clump.

☐ Substitute nonfat or low-fat cottage cheese for the cream in quiches and casseroles, replacing the cream on a measure-for-measure basis.

☐ To add extra richness to low-fat cream soups, purée some of the broth and vegetables from the soup, and return the mixture to the pot for added thickness. This will reduce the need for cream and cream substitutes.

☐ Blend $^2/_3$ cup of nonfat ricotta cheese and $^1/_3$ cup of skim milk in a blender, adding a little more milk if the resulting mixture is too thick. Use this mixture as a cream substitute in creamy sauces like Alfredo. When heating sauces made with ricotta, do *not* let them boil, or they may separate.

☐ Blend equal parts of nonfat cream cheese and skim milk in a blender until smooth, and substitute the mixture for the cream in sauces.

☐ Substitute a nonfat or light whipped topping for full-fat whipped cream in mousses, frostings, and fillings. For extra creaminess and to boost nutrition, substitute nonfat vanilla or another flavor of yogurt for a third to half of the whipped topping.

Cooking With Low-Fat and Skim Milk

Milk adds richness and body to soups and sauces, and promotes browning in baked goods. Fortunately for the low-fat cook, the low- and no-fat versions of this product can perform equally well in all your favorite dishes.

☐ Use skim or 1-percent low-fat milk to replace whole milk in any dish, from puddings, soups, and sauces, to muffins, breads, and pancakes. For extra richness, add a tablespoon of instant dry milk to each cup of skim milk.

☐ For a real treat, substitute nonfat or 1-percent low-fat buttermilk for the whole milk in muffins, breads, cakes, pancakes, waffles, and other baked goods. Buttermilk adds such a rich taste to baked goods and bread products that you'll never miss the fat.

☐ For a tangy taste and rich texture, try substituting nonfat or 1-percent low-fat buttermilk for the whole milk in mashed potatoes, sherbets and other frozen desserts, cold soups, and fruit shakes.

Cooking With Nonfat Sour Cream

Nonfat sour cream can easily replace the full-fat version in a wide range of recipes, saving you 48 grams of fat and 240 calories for each cup of full-fat sour cream that you eliminate. Here are some tips for using both this product and some healthful alternatives.

☐ Substitute nonfat sour cream for the full-fat product in salads, dips, dressings, and other cold dishes. Most brands of nonfat sour cream are also heat-stable, meaning that you can add them to sauces and gravies without fear of separation. Land O Lakes No-Fat, Breakstone's Free, and Sealtest Free are examples of brands that can be used in both hot and cold dishes.

☐ Plain nonfat yogurt is another excellent alternative to sour cream in dips, spreads, and dressings. Like some brands of nonfat sour cream, yogurt will curdle if added to hot sauces or gravies. To prevent this, first let the yogurt warm to room temperature. Then stir in 2 tablespoons of unbleached flour or 1 tablespoon of cornstarch for each cup of yogurt used. The yogurt may then be added to the sauce without fear of separation.

☐ Puréed nonfat cottage cheese is still another fine alternative to sour cream in dips, spreads, and dressings. For extra zip, add a tablespoon of lemon juice per cup of cottage cheese when puréeing.

Cooking With Fat-Free Egg Substitutes

Before there were fat-free egg substitutes, many people simply substituted egg whites for whole eggs. While this is still a good option, in some cases, egg substitutes produce better results. Just how great are your savings in cholesterol and fat when whole eggs are replaced with egg whites or a fat-free egg substitute? One large egg contains 80 calories, 5 grams of fat, and 210 milligrams of cholesterol. The equivalent amount of egg white or egg substitute contains about 30 calories, no fat, and no cholesterol. The benefits of these alternative ingredients are clear. The following guidelines will help you choose the most appropriate substitute for your dish, and enjoy the best possible results when using it.

☐ When making quiches, scrambled eggs, omelettes, frittatas, French toast, custards, puddings, and sauces, use egg substitutes for best results.

☐ When making casseroles, pancakes, waffles, and similar dishes, use egg substitutes *or* egg whites, as they will give equally good results.

☐ *Never* use egg substitute in place of whipped egg whites when making meringues, angel foods cakes, and similar dishes. Egg substitutes simply won't work in these cases.

☐ When making omelettes, frittatas, and scrambled eggs with egg substitutes, do not mix in any milk, as you might with whole eggs. Adding milk to egg substitutes weakens their texture; thus, these egg dishes will not hold together properly. Simply use the product straight from the carton.

☐ Because egg substitutes have been pasteurized (heat treated), feel free to use these products uncooked in eggnogs and salad dressings.

☐ As a general rule, substitute 3 tablespoons of fat-free egg substitute or egg white

---

Getting the Fat Out of Your Waffle Recipe or Mix

To make your favorite waffles light, crisp, and fat-free:

☐ Replace the oil in the recipe with ¾ as much buttermilk, applesauce, or other liquid.

☐ Substitute 3 egg whites for every 2 whole eggs in the recipe, and whip the egg whites to soft peaks before folding them into the batter.

☐ For an extra-crisp texture, substitute brown rice flour or cornmeal for up to half of the wheat flour. These flours add a pleasing crunch to baked goods.

---

for each whole egg. Substitute 2 tablespoons of fat-free egg substitute for 1 egg white, and 1 tablespoon of fat-free egg substitute for 1 egg yolk.

☐ When whipping up omelettes, scrambled eggs, or similar dishes, try making your own reduced-fat, reduced-cholesterol mixture from fresh eggs. As a rule of thumb, 1 whole egg plus 3 egg whites will equal the volume of 3 large eggs—and will save you 610 milligrams of cholesterol and 15 grams of fat.

Cooking With Less Oil

Though touted as being low in artery-clogging saturated fat, vegetable oils are still pure fat and are loaded with calories. Here are some ways to eliminate or reduce the oil in your recipes.

☐ Use nonstick cooking spray and a nonstick skillet for sautéing, browning, and stir-frying. If the pan becomes too dry, simply cover it for a few seconds, and the liquid from the food should add enough moisture to prevent sticking. Or add a little water, wine, or broth to the pan as needed.

☐ When making vinaigrette salad dressings, try reversing the usual proportions of 3 parts oil to 1 part vinegar. For a milder taste, replace your usual vinegar with rice vinegar, white balsamic vinegar, or raspberry vinegar.

☐ For added flavor, toss a few chopped olives into your salads, pasta dishes, and pasta sauces instead of using olive oil. A quarter cup of chopped olives has only 50 calories and 4 grams of fat, compared with a tablespoon of olive oil, which has 120 calories and 13 grams of fat.

☐ Cook with extra virgin olive oil, sesame oil, walnut oil, and similarly rich-tasting oils. These oils are so flavorful that just 2 or 3 teaspoons is often enough for a whole recipe.

☐ When you eliminate the oil or other fats from a recipe, increase the seasonings to add extra flavor. Try increasing the seasonings by 25 percent at first. Then add more if needed.

Getting the Fat Out of Your Pancake Recipe or Mix

To make fabulous fat-free pancakes using your own favorite recipe or mix, replace each tablespoon of oil in the batter with $3/4$ as much nonfat buttermilk, nonfat yogurt, applesauce, or mashed banana. For instance, if a recipe calls for 2 tablespoons of oil, substitute $1^{1}/2$ tablespoons of your chosen fat substitute. Then replace each whole egg with 3 tablespoons of fat-free egg substitute or egg white.

☐ For guidelines on replacing the oil—as well as other high-fat ingredients—in your favorite pancake and waffle recipe or mix, see the insets on pages 78 and 79.

☐ For ideas on replacing the oil in your baked goods, see the baking tips on pages 98 to 101.

Cooking With Low- and Nonfat Mayonnaise

Like full-fat margarine and butter, regular mayonnaise is a major culprit in many high-fat diets. Happily, plenty of nonfat and low-fat brands of mayonnaise are available. Here are some ideas for lightening up your recipes.

☐ Substitute nonfat or reduced-fat brands of mayonnaise for the full-fat product in tuna salads, chicken salads, cole slaw, potato salads, sauces, dressings, and many other recipes.

☐ For a super-creamy dressing that's perfect for potato, macaroni, and fruit salads, try mixing equal parts of nonfat mayonnaise and nonfat sour cream.

Cooking With Nuts

Nuts add crunch, great taste, and essential nutrients to all kinds of salads, casseroles, and baked goods. Unfortunately, nuts also add fat—about 80 grams per cup, to be exact. Here are some ideas for reducing the amount of nuts in recipes without sacrificing flavor.

☐ Toast nuts before adding them to your recipe by following the directions in the inset "Getting the Most Out of Nuts," on page 80.

☐ Finely chop nuts before adding them to recipes so that the flavor is more evenly distributed throughout the food.

☐ Instead of stirring large amounts of nuts into a recipe, use them as a garnish on salads and other dishes, or sprinkle them lightly over muffin batters before baking.

☐ Substitute Grape-Nuts cereal, toasted wheat germ, or low-fat granola for the part or all of the nuts in baked goods.

☐ When making salads, stir-fries, and similar dishes, substitute crunchy vegetables like celery, carrots, water chestnuts, and jicama for part or all of the nuts.

Getting the Most Out of Nuts

Toasting intensifies the flavor of nuts so much that you can often cut the amount used in half. Simply arrange the nuts in a single layer on a baking sheet, and bake at 350°F for about 10 minutes, or until lightly browned with a toasted, nutty smell. Be sure to check the nuts often, as once they begin to turn color, they can quickly burn. (For sliced almonds or chopped nuts, bake for only 6 to 8 minutes.) To save time, toast a large batch and store leftovers in an airtight container in the refrigerator for several weeks, or keep them in the freezer for several months.

TRIMMING THE FAT FROM MEATS

Meat—especially ground beef—is the number-one contributor of saturated fat to most people's diets. But if you know how to choose the leanest cuts (see Chapter 4), and you know a few tricks of the trade, even dishes like pot roast, tacos, and sweet and sour pork can be lightened up enough to be a part of a low-fat diet. Here are some tips for trimming the fat when purchasing and cooking meats.

☐ When purchasing beef, choose top round, eye round, round tip, and top sirloin whenever possible. Cube steaks, beef stew meat, precut stir-fry meat, and London broil are usually made from these lean cuts, and so are also good choices. Do read labels, though, as these products are sometimes made from fattier cuts, such as chuck.

☐ When eating pork, try to choose pork tenderloin, well-trimmed sirloin pork chops, and hams that are at least 95-percent lean.

☐ Choose lunchmeats that are at least 95-percent lean for sandwiches, salads, and other dishes.

☐ Substitute top round roast for brisket and for higher-fat pot roasts like chuck roast.

☐ Substitute skinless turkey breast tenderloins for veal in dishes like veal Parmesan and veal Marsala.

☐ Substitute turkey bacon for pork bacon in Southern-style vegetables, casseroles, breakfast dishes, BLT sandwiches, and salads. Canadian bacon and diced lean ham can also replace bacon in many vegetable dishes, stews, bean soups, casseroles, and other dishes.

☐ Instead of seasoning vegetables with bacon or ham, try adding Goya ham base. Located in the ethnic section of your grocery store, these ham-flavored bouillon granules add flavor without fat. Chicken or vegetable bouillon granules can serve the same purpose.

☐ Substitute 95-percent lean ground beef or ground turkey breast for higher-fat grinds of beef.

☐ Substitute fat-free or low-fat smoked sausage and kielbasa for greasy pork sausage in gumbos, jambalayas, bean soups, and casseroles. Substitute ground turkey sausage for pork sausage in breakfast casseroles and other dishes. Or try some of the low-fat vegetarian sausage alternatives.

☐ Try replacing part or all of the ground meat in tacos, chili, sloppy Joes, casseroles, burgers, meat loaves, and other dishes with one of the widely available low-fat or fat-free meat substitutes. For simple guidelines for using these products, see the inset "Cooking With Ground Meat Substitutes" on page 82.

☐ Trim all visible fat from meats before cooking. Remove the skin from poultry either before or after cooking. (There is a slight advantage to removing it before cooking.)

☐ Marinate lean cuts of meat in the refrigerator for at least 6 hours or overnight to add tenderness and flavor. (See page 89 for tips on marinating meats.)

☐ In casseroles and stir-fries, use less meat and more vegetables and grains.

☐ Use low-fat cooking techniques like grilling, broiling, stir-frying, baking, roasting, braising, stewing, oven-frying, and poaching. Pages 81 to 87 provide more details on these cooking methods.

☐ Avoid piercing meats during cooking to prevent juices from escaping.

☐ Avoid salting meats before cooking. Salt draws out moisture, making the meat dry.

COOKING TECHNIQUES THAT TRIM FAT

Many people who change over to a low-fat lifestyle find themselves baking and broiling everything. While these are excellent methods of preparing foods, many other cooking techniques can also be used to create meat, poultry, fish, and vegetable dishes with a minimum of fat and a maximum of flavor.

Baking in Parchment Paper or Aluminum Foil

With this low-fat cooking method, meat, chicken, or fish is baked inside packets of parchment paper or aluminum foil, allowing the food to cook in its own juices. This is a wonderful way to seal in natural flavor and keep foods moist *without* the use of fat.

Place a single-serving portion of the food being cooked on a square of parchment paper or foil. For added flavor, top the food with vegetables and/or seasonings and a splash of liquid, such as wine or broth. Then securely fold the parchment paper or foil to prevent leakage, and place the packets in the oven on a baking sheet. Bake fish at 450°F for about 15 minutes, or until it flakes easily with a fork. Bake meat or chicken at 350°F for about 30 minutes, or until the meat is no longer pink inside.

Blackening

With this cooking method—which is popular in many restaurants—chicken, fish, or beef is coated with a spicy blend of herbs, paprika, and pepper, and then seared in a hot

Cooking With Ground Meat Substitutes

Whether you are following a vegetarian diet or are just looking for a tasty fat-free or low-fat alternative to ground beef, meat substitutes provide a great way to replace all or part of the meat in a variety of recipes. Just follow the guidelines below for delicious results.

Frozen Meatless Crumbles

Made from soy and other vegetable proteins, fat-free products like Green Giant Harvest Burger for Recipes and Morningstar Farms Ground Meatless can be found in the freezer case of your grocery store. These products are precooked, so you simply thaw them and add them to your recipe. Use 2 cups of crumbles to replace 1 pound of ground meat. To use as a meat extender for cooked crumbled meat, mix 1 cup of thawed crumbles with 8 ounces of cooked ground meat. To use as a meat extender in burgers or meat loaves, mix 1 cup of thawed crumbles with 12 ounces to a pound of uncooked ground meat, and shape and cook as desired.

Tofu Crumbles

These mildly seasoned bits of tofu, usually found in the tofu section of the supermarket, are precooked and ready to use. Substitute one 10-ounce package—about 2 cups of crumbles—for 1 pound of cooked crumbled ground meat. To use as a meat extender for cooked crumbled meat, mix 1 cup of crumbles with 8 ounces of cooked ground meat. To use as a meat extender in burgers or meat loaves, mix 1 cup of crumbles with 12 ounces to a pound of uncooked ground meat, and shape and cook as desired.

Texturized Vegetable Protein (TVP)

Made from defatted soy flour, this product—which can be found in health foods stores and some grocery stores—comes packaged as small nuggets that you rehydrate with water. To replace 1 pound of ground meat, pour $7/8$ cup of boiling broth or water over 1 cup of TVP, and let the mixture sit for about 5 minutes, or until the liquid is absorbed. To use as a meat extender for cooked crumbled meat, rehydrate $1/2$ cup of the nuggets with 7 tablespoons of liquid, and mix the hydrated mixture with 8 ounces of cooked ground meat. To use as a meat extender in burgers or meat loaves, rehydrate $1/2$ cup of the nuggets with 7 tablespoons of liquid, mix with 12 ounces to a pound of uncooked ground meat, and shape and cook as desired.

skillet until blackened and charred on the outside, but tender and moist on the inside. Very little fat is used to cook the food. Beware, though, because melted butter or oil is sometimes poured over the food before serving. If you are in a restaurant, be sure to request that they omit the extra butter or oil. At home, of course, you can prepare blackened food with little or no fat. And since blackening seasoning can be purchased in the spice section of most grocery stores, this is an easy option for home cooking.

To blacken your chicken, fish, or lean beef at home, first coat both sides of the food with blackening seasoning. If you are blackening chicken breast halves, you will need to pound them out slightly so that they will cook quickly and evenly. Spray a nonstick skillet with nonstick cooking spray, and preheat it over medium-high heat. Then brown the food in the hot skillet until thoroughly cooked. Alternatively, coat the food with seasoning and grill or broil it according to the directions given elsewhere in this section.

Braising

A slow, moist-heat method of cooking, braising is especially well-suited to lean roasts like top round and eye round, which tend to be tough.

To braise a roast, first brown the meat on all sides in an ovenproof skillet or Dutch oven, as described on page 84. Add about $1/2$ cup of water, broth, wine, tomato juice, or another liquid and the desired seasonings to the skillet or pot. Cover tightly, and simmer over low heat on top of the stove, or bake at 300°F to 325°F until fork tender. A $2^1/2$- to 3-pound roast will take about 2 hours and 30 minutes.

If desired, add vegetables, such as potatoes, carrots, and onions, to the pot during the last 45 minutes or so of the cooking time. As the meat cooks, it will become tender and release some of its juices. These juices can then be boiled down for a few minutes to reduce the liquid into a flavorful sauce, or can be made into a savory gravy with the addition of a little flour or cornstarch. (For directions on defatting gravies and sauces, see the inset "Skimming the Fat From Cooking Liquids" on page 88.)

Broiling

Most people are familiar with this quick-and-easy technique in which food is placed on a broiler pan and cooked under an oven broiler, 4 to 6 inches beneath the heat source. Broiling is well-suited to cooking tender cuts of meat like beef top sirloin, beef tenderloin, pork loin chops, pork tenderloin, chicken, and fish. Tougher cuts like top round and London broil should always be marinated or pounded prior to broiling to insure tender results.

To retain moisture and promote browning during broiling, spray one side of the food with nonstick cooking spray, and broil that first side. Turn the food over, spray again, and finish broiling. Depending on the thickness of the meat and the desired degree of doneness, this will take 10 to 20 minutes of total cooking time. Be careful not to prick meats when broiling, as this will cause juices to seep out, resulting in a dry dish. By using a spatula or tongs rather than a fork to turn your food, you will keep it moist and juicy.

There are many ways to add flavor to broiled foods. Try coating the food with blackening seasoning, lemon pepper, or your favorite salt-free herb seasoning prior to broiling. Or brush the food with bottled nonfat or low-fat salad dressing or nonfat or low-fat mayonnaise blended with a sprinkling of herbs.

Browning

Great cooks know that browning brings out the best in foods—especially meats. Unfortunately, the traditional method of browning food often requires several table-spoons of oil, butter, or margarine. The good news is that all that extra fat is simply not necessary.

To brown meat, chicken, or vegetables with virtually no added fat, spray a thin film of nonstick cooking spray over the bottom of a nonstick skillet. Then preheat the skillet over medium-high heat, and brown the food as usual. If the food starts to stick, cover the skillet for a few seconds, and the moisture released from the food should prevent sticking. Or add a few teaspoons of water, broth, or wine. If you use both a nonstick skillet and nonstick cooking spray, it should not be necessary to add any liquid at all.

If you are browning a food that is coated with flour or crumbs, as when making chicken Parmesan, first brown one side as directed above. Then spray the top of the meat and turn it over to brown the other side. This will insure that both sides stay moist and turn golden brown.

Grilling

This popular cooking method is similar to broiling, except that the food is placed *over* a heat source rather than *under* it. The same guidelines that apply to broiling foods should be used when grilling.

Oven-Frying

A great method for cooking chicken, fish, and vegetables, this technique makes your foods crisp on the outside, and moist and tender on the inside.

First dip the chicken, fish, or vegetables in egg whites, egg substitute, yogurt, or buttermilk. Then coat the food with crushed corn flakes, dried bread crumbs, toasted wheat germ, or cornmeal. For the most flavorful results, mix the coating with poultry seasoning, paprika, lemon pepper, or Cajun seasoning.

Place the food in a single layer on a baking sheet coated with nonstick cooking spray, and spray the top lightly with cooking spray. Bake chicken at 375°F to 400°F for about 45 minutes, or until no longer pink inside. Bake fish at 400°F to 450°F for about 10 minutes, or until it flakes easily with a fork. Bake vegetables at 400°F for about 15 minutes, or until tender. Turn your oven-fried foods with a spatula about halfway through the cooking process.

Poaching

An excellent method for cooking fish and skinless chicken breasts, this technique involves cooking foods gently in a barely simmering liquid such as stock. Poaching keeps food moist and flavorful without using any fat at all.

Place your fish or chicken in a skillet or pot just large enough to permit the food to be arranged in a single layer. If you plan to use an acidic ingredient like lemon juice, wine, or tomato juice in your poaching liquid, be sure to choose nonreactive cookware, such as stainless steel, enameled steel, anodized aluminum, or glass. Cover the food with the poaching liquid of your choice, such as water or broth, adding a splash of wine or a dash of herbs for extra flavor.

Bring the liquid to a boil over medium-high heat. Then reduce the heat to low and simmer just until the food is tender. Depending on their size and thickness, fish fillets or steaks will be done in about 10 minutes. Chicken breast halves will take slightly longer. As the food poaches, flavors will be exchanged between the liquid and the food. If desired, after removing the chicken or fish, you can boil the liquid down into a flavorful sauce and serve it with the food.

Roasting

Synonymous with baking, roasting is a simple cooking method in which the food is placed in an oiled pan and cooked in an oven until done. Roasting is well-suited for cooking tender roasts like pork tenderloin and beef tenderloin, as well as poultry, fish, and even vegetables. It will leave your foods moist and tender on the inside and delightfully brown on the outside, with a deep, rich flavor.

When roasting, keep fat to a minimum by using nonstick cooking sprays rather than oil or butter. Spray it on the pan to prevent foods from sticking, and on the food itself to promote browning. When cooking beef or pork, simply season the food as desired and place it uncovered in a 350°F oven for about 20 to 35 minutes per pound, depending on the cut and the desired degree of doneness. When baking skinless poultry, it is a good idea to cover the pan with aluminum foil during the first part of the baking period to seal in moisture. Then remove the cover during the last 15 minutes to allow the food to brown. When roasting fish steaks or fillets, cook at 400°F to 450°F for about 10 minutes per inch of thickness, or until the fish flakes easily.

Roasting is also a simple and delicious way to cook vegetables. As the vegetables cook, they become tender and their natural sugars rise to the surface, caramelizing into a slightly sweet, golden coating. Most recipes for roasted vegetables call for a splash of vinegar, some herbs, and a generous amount of oil. For a healthier dish, omit all or part of the oil in the recipe, and instead toss the vegetables with a tablespoon of balsamic vinegar, some herbs, and a tablespoon of broth.

First, coat a nonstick pan with nonstick cooking spray, and arrange the vegetables in a single layer in the pan. The pan should be just large enough to hold the vegetables in one layer. (If the pan is too large, the vegetables may dry out during cooking.) If you omitted all of the oil from the recipe, spray the tops of the vegetables with some nonstick cooking spray.

For quick-cooking vegetables like eggplant, asparagus, and zucchini, roast the food uncovered at 450°F for 10 minutes. Turn with a spatula, and cook for an additional 10 minutes, or until golden and tender.

For long-cooking vegetables like carrots, potatoes, and winter squash, cover the pan with aluminum foil, and roast at 450°F for about 20 minutes. Remove the foil, and bake for 15 additional minutes. Then turn with a spatula, and roast for 15 minutes more, or until golden and tender. (Add a little broth or water to the pan during cooking if needed, but be careful not to add too much liquid or the vegetables will steam instead of roast.)

Steaming

Perfect for seafood or vegetables, steaming helps retain moisture and nutritional value in foods.

To steam your food, first place the food on a rack or in a steamer basket positioned above a liquid such as water, broth, or wine. If desired, add herbs to the steaming liquid for extra flavor. Cover the pot, and turn the heat to medium-high so that the liquid comes to a boil. Steam fish fillets and steaks for about 10 minutes per inch of thickness, and steam vegetables just until they are crisp-tender. Tender vegetables like snow peas and squash will take only a few minutes, while denser vegetables like potatoes and carrots will take longer. Be aware that you can also steam foods in a microwave oven, using a special steamer available for that purpose. Electric steamers—which can also be used to cook rice—are also available.

Because of their high water content, many vegetables can be steamed on your stovetop without any special equipment. Place cut vegetables like squash, cabbage, or sliced carrots in a large nonstick skillet. Add a small amount of water or broth and the desired seasonings, cover, and cook over medium-high heat, stirring occasionally, until tender. Vegetables like squash and spinach, which release liquid during cooking, need only a couple of tablespoons of liquid for steaming.

Stewing

This slow-cooking method is ideal for lean cuts of beef, which are tougher than higher-fat cuts. It is also a good way to cook chicken parts. Stewing gradually tenderizes the meat while retaining moisture and blending flavors.

Start with chicken parts or small pieces of meat, such as top round, eye round, and round tip. If desired, brown the meat first, following the directions on page 84. While this step will enhance the flavor, it is not necessary.

Place the meat or poultry in a large skillet or Dutch oven, and cover it with broth, water, or another liquid. Add seasonings for flavor, cover, and cook slowly over low heat for an hour to an hour and 30 minutes, or until fork tender. (Chicken parts will take only about 45 minutes.) Add any desired vegetables during the last 15 to 30 minutes of cooking to prevent them from becoming mushy. As the mixture cooks, the liquid will become a flavorful sauce that can be thickened by cooking until reduced in volume, or by the addition of a little cornstarch or flour at the end of the cooking time. (For directions on defatting the cooking liquid, see the inset "Skimming the Fat From Cooking Liquids" on page 88.)

Stir-Frying

An excellent way to cook mixtures of vegetables and meat, poultry, or tofu, stir-frying retains the foods' maximum nutritional value.

For best results, partially freeze the meat for easy slicing. Then thinly slice it across the grain. Cut the vegetables into bite-sized pieces.

Always use a nonstick skillet or wok when stir-frying, so you can cook with little or no added fat. Coat the pan with nonstick cooking spray, or use just a couple of teaspoons of vegetable oil, if desired, and preheat over medium-high heat. Add the meat, and stir-fry, continuously turning the meat with a scooping motion until it is thoroughly cooked. If the skillet becomes too dry, cover it for a few seconds and the liquid released from the meat should moisten the skillet. Or add a little broth or water to the skillet as needed.

Once the meat is fully cooked, add the longer-cooking vegetables, like carrots and broccoli, to the skillet. After a minute or 2, toss in the quick-cooking vegetables, like cabbage and bean sprouts. If you are making a large batch of stir-fry, you may need to remove the meat from the skillet or wok (cover to keep warm) while you cook the vegetables. Again, if the skillet becomes too dry, cover it briefly or add a small amount of liquid.

Return the meat to the skillet, and add a little reduced-sodium soy sauce, bottled stir-fry sauce, or other seasonings. Serve immediately.

ADDING FLAVOR WITHOUT FAT

All too many people equate fat-free cooking with *bland* cooking. But you don't have to throw out the flavor with the fat. In fact, as you learn to make healthier versions of your favorite dishes, you may discover a whole new world of aromas and flavors—herbs, spices, and condiments that add so much taste, you'll never miss the fat. Here are some ingredients that can enhance many of your favorite foods.

Vinegars, Wines, and Lemon Juice

Professional chefs routinely use small amounts of acidic liquids like vinegars, wines, and lemon juice to bring out the flavors of foods. Just a splash in soups, sauces, vegetables, meats, fish, and poultry can add the perfect finishing touch to a dish. And since acidic flavors lend the impression of saltiness, incorporating these ingredients into your recipes will reduce the need for salt. Vinegars and lemon juice can also be used as condiments at the table. Here are some ideas for using these invaluable kitchen helpers in your cooking.

☐ Squeeze some fresh lemon juice over steamed vegetables or fish.

☐ Pour a little cider vinegar over greens or green beans at the table.

☐ Dress your salad with a little red wine vinegar and a little grated Parmesan. Or, for a milder taste, try raspberry vinegar.

☐ Add a splash of malt vinegar to fish and vegetable dishes.

☐ Add a couple of tablespoons of balsamic or herb vinegar to a pot of bean soup near the end of the cooking time.

Skimming the Fat From Cooking Liquids

There are several ways to defat the liquids that develop when meats are braised, stewed, and roasted, or when they're slow-simmered to make broths. Once defatted, these flavorful liquids are practically calorie-free and ready for use in savory gravies, sauces, and soups.

☐ Refrigerate the liquid for several hours, or until the fat rises to the top and hardens. Then simply lift the fat off with a spoon and discard.

☐ When there's no time to refrigerate liquids, defat them quickly by using a fat separator cup. This handy device, which can be purchased in most grocery stores, has a specially designed spout that pours from the bottom of the cup. The fat, which floats to the top, stays in the cup.

☐ If you don't have a fat separator cup, you can easily defat your stock, cooking liquid, or pan drippings with ice cubes. Just place a few ice cubes in pot of warm—*not hot*—liquid, and let the cubes remain in the liquid for a few seconds. Then remove the cubes, as well as the fat that clings to them.

☐ Add a splash of sherry or another wine to soups and sauces.

☐ Sauté vegetables in wine instead of oil.

Mustard

This versatile low-fat condiment can enhance more than just sandwiches. Add a little mustard to your low-fat sauces, dressings, and marinades for extra flavor. Or mix with fruit juice or honey and use as a glaze for poultry. Many different kinds of mustards are available, from Dijon to Chinese to bold and spicy, so experiment with different brands.

Reduced-Sodium Soy Sauce

A couple of tablespoons of reduced-sodium soy sauce splashed into a stir-fry or marinade can add delicious flavor without fat. Beware, though—while this product has half the salt of regular soy sauce, it still provides about 500 milligrams of sodium per tablespoon.

Salsa

This zesty fat-free condiment can be used to perk up a baked potato; meat, fish, and poultry dishes; eggs; marinades; and many other foods. Since many brands of salsa contain over 200 milligrams of sodium per 2-tablespoon serving, read the labels and choose brands with the least amount of sodium.

Tabasco Sauce

Adding a few drops of Tabasco or pepper sauce to foods is a great way to enhance flavors. And like tart and sour flavors, hot flavors reduce the need for salt. In the amount normally added to foods, pepper sauce has no calories or fat and is low in sodium. So add some to dried beans, eggs, vegetables, greens, and anything else that needs a little zip!

Herbs and Spices

Herbs and spices are the very heart of fat-free cooking. Creative use of these seasonings can add a whole new dimension to foods. If you are not used to cooking with herbs and spices, have no fear. Begin simply, by using a variety of preblended herb and spice mixtures, such as Cajun seasoning, Italian seasoning, lemon pepper, and commercial salt-free seasoning blends. Then gradually start experimenting with other herbs and spices.

The table that begins on page 90 will guide you in choosing the herbs, spices, and other flavorings that will best complement the flavor of the food you're making. Select one or two of the seasonings from the list, and try them in your dish. How much should you add to your recipe? Start with 1 to 2 teaspoons of dried herbs (or 1 to 2 tablespoons of fresh herbs) for 1 pound of meat, 4 cups of vegetables, or 4 cups of cooked pasta, rice, or grain. Then add more to taste.

Marinades and Rubs

Any steak lover will tell you that fat adds tenderness and flavor to meats. While this may be true, marinades and rubs are far more healthful and interesting ways to enhance the taste of meats—and of seafood and poultry, too. In addition, marinades help tenderize meats.

Marinades

A marinade is a seasoned liquid that is used to tenderize and add flavor to a food. Lean cuts of beef, like top round and eye round, which tend to be tough, should always be marinated if they are going to be broiled or grilled. (If these cuts are going to be braised or stewed, marinating is not necessary.) Marinades also make other cuts of beef, as well as pork and chicken, deliciously tender, and can be used to add flavor to tofu and seafood, as well.

Marinades typically contain oil; seasonings; and an acidic ingredient such as lemon or lime juice, wine, tomato juice, fruit juice, yogurt, or buttermilk. As the meat marinates, the acid ingredient acts as a tenderizer and the seasonings impart flavor. Oil is not a necessary ingredient in marinades, and can be replaced by broth or another liquid.

For a marinade to be an effective meat tenderizer, the meat must remain in the liquid for at least six hours. (An exception is seafood, which is generally not marinated for more than an hour to prevent the acid from "cooking" the fish.) Be sure to place the meat and marinade in a nonreactive container—one made of glass, plastic, or stainless steel, for instance—and refrigerate for the desired length of time. A word

A Guide to Complementary Seasonings

Food	Suggested Seasonings
Asparagus	Dill weed, lemon juice or rind, lemon pepper, mustard, tarragon, thyme, white balsamic vinegar, white wine vinegar.
Beans and peas	Balsamic vinegar, bay leaf, celery seed, chili powder, cilantro, coriander, cumin, garlic, herb vinegar, marjoram, mustard, onion, paprika, pepper sauce, sage, savory, thyme, wine vinegar.
Beef	Balsamic vinegar, bay leaf, Cajun seasoning, celery seed, chili powder, curry powder, garlic, horseradish, Italian seasoning, marjoram, onions, oregano, red wine, sage, thyme.
Broccoli	Dill weed, lemon juice or rind, lemon pepper, mustard.
Brussels sprouts	Dill seed, lemon juice or rind, lemon pepper, mustard, thyme, vinegar.
Cabbage	Caraway seed, celery seed, cider vinegar, mustard.
Carrots	Caraway seed, cardamom, dill weed, lemon, lemon pepper, mace, marjoram, nutmeg, parsley.
Cauliflower	Curry, dill weed, marjoram, mustard, rosemary, tarragon.
Corn	Chili powder, cilantro, cumin, onion, red and green bell pepper.
Cucumbers	Chives, dill seed, dill weed, onion, seasoned rice vinegar, white wine vinegar.
Eggplant	Basil, garlic, Italian seasoning, marjoram, oregano, thyme.
Fish and seafood	Cajun seasoning, chervil, curry, dill weed, dill seed, garlic, ginger, lemon juice, lemon pepper, malt vinegar, mustard, onion, rosemary, saffron, tarragon, thyme, white balsamic vinegar, white wine.
Green beans	Balsamic vinegar, basil, cider vinegar, dill seed, Italian seasoning, lemon rind or juice, marjoram, mushrooms, mustard, onion, pepper sauce, savory, thyme, white wine vinegar.

Food	Suggested Seasonings
Greens, cooked	Cider vinegar, garlic, pepper sauce.
Lima beans	Onion, sage, savory, thyme.
Mushrooms	Balsamic vinegar, garlic, Italian seasoning, marjoram, sherry, red or white wine, thyme.
Noodles and pasta	Dill weed, parsley, poppy seeds, saffron.
Peas	Basil, marjoram, mint, rosemary, thyme.
Pork	Allspice, balsamic vinegar, bay leaf, Cajun seasoning, caraway, fennel, ginger, lemon pepper, mustard, onions, orange rind, oregano, rosemary, sage, sherry, thyme, white wine.
Potatoes	Chives, dill weed, garlic, onion, parsley.
Poultry	Allspice, Cajun seasoning, curry, garlic, ginger, Italian seasoning, lemon pepper, marjoram, mustard, onions, paprika, rosemary, saffron, sage, savory, sherry, tarragon, thyme, white balsamic vinegar, white wine, white wine vinegar.
Rice	Curry, mushrooms, onions, parsley, saffron, turmeric.
Salads	Basil, garlic, garlic vinegar, herb vinegar, Italian seasoning, lemon juice, oregano, raspberry vinegar, red or white wine vinegar.
Spinach	Cider vinegar, garlic, herb vinegar, lemon juice or rind, nutmeg.
Squash, summer	Basil, chives, dill weed, Italian seasoning, parsley, savory.
Squash, winter	Allspice, cardamom, cinnamon, ginger, nutmeg, orange rind.
Sweet potatoes	Allspice, cardamom, cinnamon, cloves, nutmeg, orange rind.
Tomatoes	Basil, chives, herb vinegar, Italian seasoning, marjoram, oregano, red wine vinegar, thyme.

of caution is in order. Do not marinate meats for longer than twenty-four hours, as the meat fibers on the outside of the cut can become mushy.

If, after removing the meat from the marinade, you want to use any of the left-over liquid for a sauce, always bring it to a rolling boil for at least one minute before serving. To use the marinade as a basting sauce during cooking, you must also first bring it to a rolling boil for at least one minute. Be careful not to contaminate fully cooked meats or poultry by adding sauce with a brush that was used on raw or under-cooked foods.

Rubs

A rub is a mixture of herbs and spices—and sometimes other ingredients—that is used to coat the surface of tender cuts of meat like beef sirloin and tenderloin, pork loin chops and pork tenderloin, chicken, and fish. A rub can be either a dry mixture of herbs and spices or a paste made of herbs, spices, and ingredients like crushed fresh garlic, finely chopped onions, mustard, and/or a small amount of soy sauce, vinegar, lemon or lime juice, or other liquid. Create your own blend of ingredients, use a ready-made blend such as lemon pepper or blackening seasoning, or try the recipes on page 93.

To apply the rub, first rinse the food and pat it dry with paper towels. Then, using your fingers, rub the outside surface of the meat with the seasoning blend. Let the food sit at room temperature for 30 minutes to an hour before cooking to allow the seasonings to permeate the food. (Refrigerate if you are going to let the food sit for more than an hour.) Spray the food lightly with nonstick cooking spray, and then grill, broil, or roast the food—and enjoy great flavor without added fat!

BAKING WITHOUT FAT

Contrary to popular belief, most baked goods get far more calories from fat than from sugar. Those ingredients that are the very worst culprits are cooking oils and shortenings such as butter and margarine. Fortunately, these fat-budget busters—as well as chocolate, eggs, and other high-fat ingredients—can be easily replaced with more healthful alternatives. Let's learn about the substitutions and other fat-saving tricks that will let you have your cake and eat it, too.

Substitute Other Ingredients for Fat

Almost any moist ingredient can replace the fat in muffins, breads, biscuits, cakes, brownies, and many other baked goods. It is important to realize, though, that some recipes are better candidates for fat reduction than others. So when you modify your recipes, start by eliminating only half the fat at first. Evaluate the results, then gradually reduce the amount of fat in the recipe each time you make it until you find the lowest level of fat that will produce the results you desire. Many baked goods can be made totally fat-free. Quick breads, muffins, chocolate cakes, brownies, and carrot cakes are among the easiest recipes to defat. You may be able to replace only half the fat in cakes that are meant to be very light and tender, and in biscuits, pastries, and crisp-textured cookies.

Flavorful Rubs and Marinades

Bursting with flavor, rubs and marinades can transform bland and boring meat, seafood, and poultry into delicious culinary creations. When time is in short supply, rubs are just what you need to perk up a meal. Use a commercial premixed blend like Cajun seasoning, or make your own mixture using one of the following recipes. When you have more time, make use of marinades. These mixtures are especially good when preparing lean cuts of meat, which are often tough, as the marinades add tenderness as well as fabulous flavor.

Spicy Tex-Mex Rub

Yield: $^1/_4$ cup, or enough for about 2 pounds of meat

1 tablespoon chili powder
1 tablespoon dark brown sugar
2 teaspoons lemon pepper

1 teaspoon ground cumin
$^1/_2$ teaspoon garlic powder
$^1/_4$ teaspoon salt

1. Combine all of the ingredients in a small bowl, and stir to mix well.

2. Apply the rub to your choice of meat, seafood, or poultry according to the directions on page 92. Then grill, broil, or roast the food as desired.

NUTRITIONAL FACTS (PER 2-TEASPOON SERVING)
Calories: 15 Carbohydrates: 3.1 g Cholesterol: 0 mg
Fat: 0.2 g Fiber: 0.5 g Protein: 0.2 g Sodium: 47 mg

Rosemary Rub

Yield: $^1/_4$ cup, or enough for about 2 pounds of meat

2 tablespoons dried rosemary
1 tablespoon dried grated lemon rind
1 tablespoon light brown sugar
$^3/_4$ teaspoon coarsely ground black
  pepper

$^3/_4$ teaspoon garlic powder
$^1/_4$ teaspoon salt
1 tablespoon prepared mustard

1. Combine all of the ingredients except for the mustard in a small bowl, and stir to mix well. Add the mustard, and stir until the mixture forms a thick paste.

2. Apply the rub to your choice of meat, seafood, or poultry according to the directions on page 92. Then grill, broil, or roast the food as desired.

NUTRITIONAL FACTS (PER 2-TEASPOON SERVING)
Calories: 13 Carbohydrates: 2.8 g Cholesterol: 0 mg
Fat: 0.2 g Fiber: 0.5 g Protein: 0.3 g Sodium: 122 mg

Teriyaki Marinade

Yield: ³/4 cup, or enough for 2 pounds of meat

¹/2 cup orange juice

3 tablespoons reduced-sodium
   soy sauce

2 tablespoons dark brown sugar

1 teaspoon crushed fresh garlic

³/4 teaspoon ground ginger

1. Combine all of the ingredients in a small bowl, and stir to mix well.

2. Marinate your choice of meat, seafood, or poultry according to the directions on page 89. Then grill, broil, or roast the food as desired.

NUTRITIONAL FACTS (PER SERVING)
Calories: 14 Carbohydrates: 3.1 g Cholesterol: 0 mg
Fat: 0 g Fiber: 0 g Protein: 0.4 g Sodium: 127 mg

Lemon-Herb Marinade

Yield: ³/8 cup, or enough for 2 pounds of meat

¹/4 cup lemon juice

2 tablespoons dark brown sugar

2 teaspoons crushed fresh garlic

2 teaspoons dried oregano, rosemary, or thyme

1 teaspoon ground black pepper

¹/2 teaspoon salt

1. Combine all of the ingredients in a small bowl, and stir to mix well.

2. Marinate your choice of meat, seafood, or poultry according to the directions on page 89. Then grill, broil, or roast the food as desired.

NUTRITIONAL FACTS (PER SERVING)
Calories: 7 Carbohydrates: 1.9 g Cholesterol: 0 mg
Fat: 0 g Fiber: 0 g Protein: 0 g Sodium: 89 mg

Be aware that reduced-fat baked goods will cook faster than their full-fat counterparts. By reducing the oven temperature and/or cooking time according to the guidelines in the tables on pages 98 through 101, you can insure that your baked goods will turn out moist and flavorful—not dry and tasteless. And, finally, to get the best results in your fat-free and low-fat baked goods, it is best to substitute whole wheat pastry flour or oat flour for at least a third of the white flour, or to substitute oat bran for a fourth of the white flour. Not only do these products add fiber and nutrients, but they also help maintain a pleasing texture. (Read more about these products on pages 61 and 62.)

Trimming the Fat From Made-From-Mix Baked Goods

Any of your favorite commercial cake, brownie, muffin, quick bread, and cookie mixes can be made without the usual oil or butter, allowing you to cut the fat in these products by up to 75 percent. Before making any changes in the recipe, check the package directions, as many manufacturers offer guidelines for mixing up the product without oil alongside the regular directions. If no low-fat directions are offered, use the following guidelines.

Cake, Quick Bread, and Muffin Mixes

Choose a fat substitute that will complement the flavor of your mix. For instance, use applesauce in yellow cakes, nonfat sour cream in white cakes and blueberry muffins, mashed bananas in spice cakes and banana bread, and applesauce or Prune Purée (page 102) in chocolate cakes. Then use these guidelines for replacing the butter, oil, and eggs in the recipe:

☐ Replace the butter in mixes with half as much fat substitute.

☐ Replace the oil with three-fourths as much fat substitute.

☐ Replace each egg with 3 tablespoons of fat-free egg substitute or egg white.

☐ Check the product for doneness several minutes before the end of the usual baking time, and be careful not to overbake.

☐ If the product seems too dry, use more fat substitute next time. (Some mixes will require a one-for-one substitution of fat substitute for butter or oil.)

Brownie Mixes

Again, choose a fat substitute that will complement the flavor of your mix. Applesauce, mashed bananas, and Prune Purée (page 102) are all good choices for brownies. Then use these guidelines for replacing the butter, oil, and eggs in the recipe:

☐ Replace the butter in mixes with half as much fat substitute.

☐ Replace the oil with three-fourths as much fat substitute.

☐ Replace each egg with 3 tablespoons of fat-free egg substitute or egg white.

☐ Check the product for doneness several minutes before the end of the usual baking time, and be careful not to overbake.

☐ Note that a one-for-one substitution of fat substitute for fat is usually not needed for brownie mixes. Adding more fat substitute than is necessary will most likely give the brownies a cake-like texture, rather than a chewy, fudgy texture.

Cookie Mixes

When trimming the fat from made-from-mix cookies, you'll have best results using one of these three fat substitutes: homemade Prune Purée (page 102), or the commercial products Sunsweet Lighter Bake or Wonderslim. Then follow these guidelines to replace the oil, solid shortening, and eggs in the recipe.

☐ Replace the oil with three-fourths as much Prune Purée, Sunsweet Lighter Bake, or WonderSlim fat substitute.

☐ Replace the butter, margarine, or other solid shortening in mixes with half as much Prune Purée, Sunsweet Lighter Bake, or WonderSlim fat substitute.

☐ Replace each egg with 2 tablespoons of Prune Purée, Sunsweet Lighter Bake, or WonderSlim fat substitute, or with 2 tablespoons of water.

☐ Spray the cookie sheet with nonstick cooking spray (even if the directions say to use an ungreased sheet), and flatten the cookie dough slightly with the tip of a spoon before baking to facilitate spreading.

☐ Bake the cookies for the directed amount of time and at the recommended oven temperature, or until golden brown.

Bake With Reduced-Fat Margarine and Light Butter

Contrary to popular belief, reduced-fat margarine and light butter *can* be substituted for their full-fat counterparts in many baked goods. These products make it possible to reduce fat by more than half, and still enjoy light, tender, buttery tasting cakes; crisp cookies; flaky pie crusts; and other goodies that are not easily made fat-free. Use the following guidelines as a starting point when making substitutions:

☐ Because reduced-fat margarine and butter are diluted with water, they cannot be substituted for regular butter and margarine on a one-for-one basis. To compensate for the extra water, substitute three-fourths of the light product for the full-fat butter or margarine. For instance, if a cake recipe calls for 1 cup of butter, use ³/₄ cup of light butter.

☐ For best results, use a brand that contains 5 to 6 grams of fat and 50 calories per tablespoon. (Full-fat brands contain 11 grams of fat and 100 calories per tablespoon.) Brands with less fat than this will work in some, but not all, baked goods.

☐ Be careful not to overbake your reduced-fat creations, as they can become dry. Reduce the oven temperature by 25°F, and check the product for doneness a few minutes before the end of the usual baking time.

Substitute Oil for Butter and Margarine

Another good way to reduce the fat in baked goods is to replace the butter, margarine, or other solid shortening with half as much oil.

This technique will make it possible to create moist and tender cakes, breads, and biscuits; crisp cookies; and tender pie crusts—all with half the original fat. When making this substitution, try using walnut oil for a nutty flavor or unrefined corn oil for a buttery flavor. Or add a little butter-flavored extract to your dough or batter. Bake as usual, checking the product for doneness a few minutes before the end of the recommended baking time.

Substitute Cocoa Powder for Chocolate

By substituting cocoa powder for baking chocolate, you will save 111 calories and 13.5 grams of fat for each ounce of baking chocolate called for. How can you replace chocolate with a powder? Simply use 3 tablespoons of cocoa powder plus 1 tablespoon of water or another liquid for each ounce of baking chocolate in cakes, brownies, cookies, muffins, and other goodies. Here are some other tips for chocolate lovers.

☐ For the deepest, darkest, richest cocoa flavor, use Dutch processed cocoa in your chocolate treats. Dutching, a process that neutralizes the natural acidity in cocoa, results in a darker, sweeter, more mellow-flavored cocoa. Look for a brand like Hershey's Dutch Processed European Style cocoa. Like regular cocoa, this product has only half a gram of fat per tablespoon—although some brands do contain more fat. Dutched cocoa can be substituted for regular cocoa in any recipe, and since it has a smoother, sweeter flavor, you may find that you can reduce the sugar in your recipe by up to 25 percent.

☐ Replace the butter, margarine, or shortening in your chocolate treats with Prune Butter (page 102). Sweet, nutritious, and fat-free, Prune Butter adds moistness to baked goods and enhances the flavor of chocolate. You will never miss the fat!

Using Fat Substitutes in Cookies and Brownies

Fat Substitutes	In Which Items Do These Work Best?	How Should Your Recipes Be Modified When Using These Fat Substitutes?
Applesauce, mashed banana, puréed fruits, nonfat or low-fat buttermilk, and nonfat yogurt.	Use applesauce, buttermilk, or yogurt when you want to change the taste as little as possible. Use mashed bananas, puréed raspberries, and other fruits for a change of pace.	• Replace part or all of the butter, margarine, or other solid fat in brownies with ½ as much fat substitute. Replace part or all of the oil with ¾ as much fat substitute. Mix up the batter, and add more substitute if the batter seems too dry. • Using the same guidelines, replace up to half the fat in cookie recipes. • Replace each egg in brownie and cookie recipes with 3 tablespoons of fat-free egg substitute, if desired. • Bake reduced-fat brownies at 325°F, and check for doneness a few minutes before the end of the usual baking time. Remove the brownies from the oven as soon as the edges are firm and the center is almost set. • Bake reduced-fat cookies at 275°F to 300°F, and bake for 15 to 20 minutes, or until lightly browned.
Honey, maple syrup, molasses, corn syrup, Fruit Source liquid, chocolate syrup, fruit jams and spreads, and fruit juice concentrates.	Use honey or fruit jam in oatmeal cookies; chocolate syrup in brownies; and maple syrup or molasses in spice cookies. Use corn syrup and Fruit Source liquid when you want to change the taste as little as possible. Use fruit juice concentrates in oatmeal and spice cookies.	• Replace part or all of the butter, margarine, or other solid fat in cookies and brownies with ¾ as much fat substitute. Replace part or all of the oil with an equal amount of fat substitute. Mix up the batter, and add more substitute if the batter seems too dry. Note that totally fat-free cookies will be chewy in texture. If you want crisp cookies, replace no more than half the fat. • Replace each whole egg in cookie recipes with 3 tablespoons of fat-free egg substitute or 2 tablespoons of water if desired. Replace each egg in brownie recipes with 3 tablespoons of fat-free egg substitute, if desired. • Reduce the sugar in cookie and brownie recipes by the amount of fat substitute being added. • Bake reduced-fat brownies at 325°F, and check for doneness a few minutes before the end of the usual baking time. Remove the brownies from the oven as soon as the edges are firm and the center is almost set. • Bake reduced-fat cookies at 275°F to 300°F. Bake for 15 to 20 minutes, or until lightly browned.

Fat Substitutes	In Which Items Do These Work Best?	How Should Your Recipes Be Modified When Using These Fat Substitutes?
Prune Butter (page 102)	This substitute is delicious in brownies and in spice, oatmeal, and chocolate cookies.	• Replace part or all of the butter, margarine, or other solid fat in brownies and cookies with an equal amount of fat substitute. • Replace each whole egg in brownie and cookie recipes with 3 tablespoons of fat-free egg substitute, if desired. • Reduce the sugar in cookie and brownie recipes by $1/2$ to $2/3$ the amount of fat substitute. • Bake reduced-fat brownies at 325°F, and check for doneness a few minutes before the end of the baking time. Remove from the oven as soon as edges are firm and center is almost set. • Bake reduced-fat cookies at 350°F, and check for doneness a few minutes before the end of the usual baking time.
Prune Purée (page 102)	Because of Prune Purée's mild flavor, it works well in all recipes.	• Replace part or all of the butter, margarine, or other solid fat in cookies and brownies with $1/2$ as much Prune Purée. Replace part or all of the oil with $3/4$ as much of the purée. • Replace each whole egg in brownie recipes with three tablespoons of egg substitute, if desired. Replace each whole egg in cookie recipes with one egg white or two additional tablespoons of Prune Purée. • Bake reduced-fat brownies at 325°F, and check for doneness a few minutes before end of baking time. Remove from the oven as soon as edges are firm and center is almost set. • Bake reduced-fat cookies at 350°F, and check for doneness a few minutes before end of baking time.
Mashed cooked or canned pumpkin, butternut squash, and sweet potatoes	Use any of these substitutes in oatmeal, spice, and chocolate cookie recipes, and in brownies.	• Replace part or all of the butter or margarine in brownies with $1/2$ to $3/4$ as much fat substitute. Replace part or all of the oil with $3/4$ as much fat substitute. Add more substitute if batter seems dry. • Using the same guidelines, replace up to $1/2$ the fat in cookie recipes. • Replace each egg in cookie and brownie recipes with 3 tablespoons of egg substitute, if desired. • Bake reduced-fat brownies at 325°F, and check for doneness a few minutes before end of baking time. Remove from the oven as soon as edges are firm and center is almost set. • Bake reduced-fat cookies at 275°F to 300°F, and check for doneness a few minutes before end of baking time.

Using Fat Substitutes in Muffins, Quick Breads, and Cakes

Fat Substitutes	In Which Items Do These Work Best?	How Should Your Recipes Be Modified When Using These Fat Substitutes?
Applesauce, mashed banana, puréed fruits, fruit juice, nonfat or low-fat buttermilk, nonfat yogurt, and skim milk.	Use applesauce, non-fat or low-fat butter-milk, nonfat yogurt, or skim milk to make biscuits, muffins, chocolate cakes, and other baked goods whose flavor you do not want to change. Use fruit juices and purées in carrot and spice cakes, breads, and muffins.	• Replace part or all of the butter, margarine, or other solid fat in muffins, breads, biscuits, scones, and cakes with 1/2 as much of the chosen fat substitute. Replace part or all of the oil with 3/4 as much fat substitute. Mix up the batter, and add more substitute if the batter seems too dry. • Replace each whole egg with one egg white. • Reduce the oven temperature by 25°F. • Check for doneness a few minutes before the end of the usual baking time.
Honey, maple syrup, corn syrup, chocolate syrup, fruit jams and spreads, and fruit juice concentrates.	Use honey or fruit jam in muffins; maple syrup in spice cakes and muffins; fruit juice concentrates in muffins and breads; corn syrup in white cakes and other baked goods whose flavor you do not want to change; and chocolate syrup in chocolate cakes and other chocolate treats.	• Replace part or all of the butter, margarine, or other solid fat in muffins, breads, scones, and cakes with 3/4 as much fat substitute. Replace part or all of the oil with an equal amount of fat substitute. Mix up the batter, and add more substitute if the batter seems too dry. • Replace each whole egg with one egg white. • Reduce the sugar by the amount of fat substitute being added. • Reduce the oven temperature by 25°F. • Check for doneness a few minutes before the end of the usual baking time.
Prune Butter (page 102)	This substitute is delicious in chocolate cakes and in fruit- or spice-flavored muffins, breads, and cakes.	• Replace part or all of the butter, margarine, or other solid fat in muffins, breads, scones, and cakes with an equal amount of Prune Butter. • Replace each whole egg with one egg white. • Reduce the sugar by 1/2 to 2/3 the amount of Prune Butter being added. • Reduce the oven temperature by 25°F. • Check for doneness a few minutes before the end of the usual baking time.

Fat Substitutes	In Which Items Do These Work Best?	How Should Your Recipes Be Modified When Using These Fat Substitutes?
Prune Purée (page 102)	Because of Prune Purée's mild flavor, it works well in all recipes.	• Replace part or all of the butter, margarine, or other solid fat in muffins, breads, scones, and cakes with 1/2 as much Prune Purée. Replace part or all of the oil with 3/4 as much of the purée. Mix up the batter, and add more substitute if the batter seems too dry. • Replace each whole egg with one egg white or two additional tablespoons of Prune Purée. • Reduce the oven temperature by 25°F. • Check for doneness a few minutes before the end of the usual baking time.
Mashed cooked or canned pumpkin, butternut squash, and sweet potatoes.	Use these substitutes in biscuits, muffins, breads, and spice cakes. They work particularly well in citrus- and pineapple-flavored baked goods.	• Replace part or all of the butter, margarine, or other solid fat in muffins, breads, scones, biscuits, and cakes with 3/4 as much fat substitute. Replace part or all of the oil with an equal amount of fat substitute. Mix up the batter, and add more substitute if the batter seems too dry. • Replace each whole egg with one egg white. • Reduce the oven temperature by 25°F. • Check for doneness a few minutes before the end of the usual baking time.

Use Egg Substitutes and Egg Whites Instead of Whole Eggs

Replace each whole egg in your low-fat baked goods with 3 tablespoons of fat-free egg substitute or egg white. To add extra lightness and tenderness to low-fat and fat-free cakes, muffins, and quick breads, beat some of the egg whites to soft peaks and fold them into the prepared batter.

Choose the Right Flours for Fat-Free and Low-Fat Baking

Fat is an essential ingredient in baked goods because it interferes with the development of gluten, the protein in wheat flour that can cause a tough, coarse texture when batters are overmixed. Therefore, when eliminating the fat from baked goods, it is important to use a low-gluten flour and to stir or beat the batter just until it is well mixed. Whole wheat pastry flour is an excellent choice for baking because it is low in gluten, and it also contains fiber, which interferes with gluten development. Baked goods made with whole wheat pastry flour will be lighter and more tender than those made with refined white flour. Many fat-free recipes call for cake flour, which is also low in gluten. However, cake flour, which is highly refined and processed with chlorine gas, is not a nutritious choice.

Making Prune Butter and Prune Purée

As you have seen, a variety of fat substitutes—including applesauce, baby food fruits, puréed fruits, nonfat sour cream, and nonfat buttermilk—can replace the fat in baked goods. These products are readily available in grocery stores. Two additional substitutes, Prune Butter and Prune Purée, not only can be found on grocery store shelves, but can easily be made at home.

Prune Butter

This sweet, nutritious, fiber-rich fat substitute works beautifully in brownies and other chocolate treats, as well as in spice cakes. And the jam and jelly section of most grocery stores stocks at least one type of Prune Butter, such as Levkar Prune Butter or Solo Prune Plum Filling.

If you would prefer to use a homemade product, you'll find that it's easy to whip up your own Prune Butter. To make 1 cup, combine 8 ounces (about 1 1/3 cups) of pitted prunes with 6 tablespoons of water in a food processor, and process into a smooth paste. Prune Butter keeps beautifully for up to three weeks when refrigerated in an airtight container. You can also freeze Prune Butter for several months.

Prune Purée

Like Prune Butter, Prune Purée works well in a variety of baked goods. When you don't have time to whip up your own Prune Purée, look for WonderSlim fat substitute. A nutritious product, it can be found in many health foods and grocery stores. Another ready-made alternative to homemade Prune Purée is Sunsweet Lighter Bake, which can be found in the baking section of many grocery stores.

Like Prune Butter, Prune Purée is a snap to make at home. For 1 1/2 cups of Prune Purée, combine 3 ounces (about 1/2 cup) of pitted prunes, 1 cup of water, and 2 teaspoons of lecithin granules* in a blender or food processor, and process until smooth. Store Prune Purée in the refrigerator for up to three weeks, or keep it in the freezer for several months.

*Lecithin, a nutritious food supplement, is sold in most health foods stores.

You can also improve the texture of fat-free and low-fat baked goods by substituting oat flour or oat bran for a quarter to a third of the refined white flour in recipes. Since oats are low in gluten, they will help maintain a tender texture. The soluble fiber in oats will also help retain moisture in your fat-free and low-fat baked goods.

Chapter 4 presents more information on these whole grain flours, and the following guidelines will allow you to substitute various whole grain flours for refined flours in your own favorite recipes.

1 cup refined wheat flour equals:

☐ 1 cup unbleached flour

☐ 1 cup whole wheat pastry flour

☐ 1 cup minus 1 tablespoon white whole wheat flour

☐ 1 cup minus 2 tablespoons regular whole wheat flour

☐ 1 cup minus 2 tablespoons brown rice flour

☐ 1 cup oat flour

☐ 1 cup barley flour

Reduce the Amount of Coconut Used in Recipes

Sprinkle just a little coconut over the tops of cakes, muffins, and other baked goods, rather than adding large amounts of this high-fat ingredient to batters. For extra flavor, add a little coconut-flavored extract to the batter.

Reduce the Amount of Nuts in Recipes

See page 80 for tips on getting the most out of nuts.

The products and techniques now available to slash the fat from virtually any dish are truly astounding in number, and, in most cases, are simple to use. In the next chapter, you'll see these techniques put into practice in fifty tantalizing recipes for appetizers, soups, salads, entrées, and more. You'll be delighted to find that eating delicious, satisfying foods is just another secret of living fat-free.

6. Recipes for Living Fat-Free

Chapters 4 and 5 provided plenty of ideas for choosing and using the best low and no-fat ingredients available. But the proof is in the pudding, so this chapter puts these principles into practice by providing fifty taste-tempting recipes that will deliciously fit into your low-fat lifestyle. As you will see, low-fat cooking does not have to be a complicated ordeal that uses every pan in the kitchen. Nor do you have to give up family favorites like pot roast with sour cream gravy, crisp fried chicken, and hearty southwestern omelettes.

Because a healthful diet is more than just low in fat, these recipes take low-fat eating one step further. Fiber-rich whole grains and whole grain flours, as well as vegetables, fruits, and legumes, are featured in plentiful amounts to help you follow all of the guidelines for good eating presented in Chapter 2. Whenever possible, natural sweeteners like fruits and juices are included to reduce the need for added sugar. And the skillful use of herbs, spices, and seasonings helps the sodium count remain low.

So that you know exactly what you are getting, each recipe includes a nutritional analysis along with an estimate of the calories and fat grams you save by using low- and no-fat products. This analysis is based on a comparison of the low-fat recipe with a standard recipe that uses full-fat ingredients.

The recipes on the following pages will show you that any dish, from appetizers to desserts, can be made delicious and satisfying without being rich and fattening. So eat well and enjoy! It is possible to do both—at every meal of the day, and on every day of the year.

PLEASING APPETIZERS & HORS D'OEUVRES

Chicken Fingers With Honey Mustard Sauce

Yield: 20 appetizers

3 cups corn flakes

$1/2$ teaspoon poultry seasoning

$1/4$ teaspoon ground black pepper

3 tablespoons fat-free egg substitute

3 tablespoons skim milk

1 pound boneless skinless chicken breasts (about 4 breast halves)

Nonstick cooking spray

SAUCE

$1/4$ cup plus 2 tablespoons nonfat or reduced-fat mayonnaise

3 tablespoons spicy mustard

3 tablespoons honey

2 tablespoons lemon juice

1. Place the corn flakes in a blender or food processor, and process into crumbs. (You should get about $3/4$ cup of crumbs. Adjust the amount if necessary.)

2. Combine the corn flake crumbs, poultry seasoning, and pepper in a shallow dish. Stir to mix well, and set aside.

3. Combine the egg substitute and milk in a shallow dish. Stir to mix well, and set aside.

4. Cut each chicken breast half into 5 long strips. Dip each strip first in the egg mixture, and then in the crumb mixture, turning to coat each side with the crumbs.

5. Coat a large baking sheet with nonstick cooking spray, and arrange the strips in a single layer on the sheet. Spray the tops of the strips lightly with cooking spray, and bake at 400°F for 15 minutes, or until the strips are golden brown and no longer pink inside.

6. While the chicken is baking, place all of the sauce ingredients in a small dish, and stir to mix well. Arrange the chicken strips on a serving platter, and serve hot, accompanied by the bowl of sauce.

NUTRITIONAL FACTS (PER APPETIZER, WITH 2 TEASPOONS OF SAUCE)
Calories: 51   Carbohydrates: 6 g   Cholesterol: 13 mg
Fat: 0.4 g   Fiber: 0.1 g   Protein: 5.8 g   Sodium: 111 mg

You Save: Calories: 35   Fat: 5 g

Savory Spinach Dip

Yield: 4 cups

1 package (10 ounces) frozen chopped spinach, thawed and squeezed dry

2 cups nonfat sour cream

1/2 cup nonfat or reduced-fat mayonnaise

1 can (8 ounces) sliced water chestnuts, drained and chopped

1/2 cup thinly sliced scallions

1 package (1 1/2 ounces) dry vegetable soup mix

1. Combine all of the ingredients in a large bowl, and stir to mix well. Cover the dip, and chill for several hours.

2. Serve in a hollowed-out round loaf of pumpernickel, accompanied by raw vegetables and whole grain crackers. Or use as a filling for finger sandwiches or hollowed-out cherry tomatoes.

NUTRITIONAL FACTS (PER TABLESPOON)

Calories: 13   Carbohydrates: 2.5 g   Cholesterol: 0 mg
Fat: 0 g   Fiber: 0.3 g   Protein: 0.7 g   Sodium: 35 mg

You Save: Calories: 27   Fat: 3.9 g

Mexican Bean Dip

Yield: About 2 1/2 cups

1 can (15 ounces) pinto beans, rinsed and drained

1/4 cup nonfat sour cream

2–3 teaspoons chili powder

1/2 teaspoon ground cumin

1/2 cup shredded nonfat or reduced-fat Cheddar cheese

1/4 cup thinly sliced scallions

1/4 cup sliced black olives

2 tablespoons finely chopped jalapeño peppers

1. Place the beans, sour cream, chili powder, and cumin in the bowl of a food processor, and process until smooth. Spread the mixture over the bottom of a 9-inch glass pie pan. Top with the cheese, followed by the scallions, olives, and jalapeños.

2. Serve at room temperature or hot. If serving hot, cook in a microwave oven at high power for about 5 minutes, or until the edges are bubbly and the cheese is melted. Or bake in a conventional oven at 400°F for about 20 minutes. Serve with baked tortilla chips.

NUTRITIONAL FACTS (PER TABLESPOON)
Calories: 14   Carbohydrates: 2.1 g   Cholesterol: 0 mg
Fat: 0.1 g   Fiber: 0.7 g   Protein: 1.2 g   Sodium: 44 mg

You Save: Calories: 11   Fat: 2 g

Hot Artichoke Appetizers

Yield: 40 appetizers

3 packages (10 ounces each) frozen
  artichoke hearts, thawed, or 3 cans
  (14 ounces each) artichoke hearts,
  drained

5 slices ham (at least 97% lean),
  4 inches square each (1 ounce each)

MARINADE
^{1}/₃ cup Dijon mustard

^{1}/₃ cup water

^{1}/₄ cup finely chopped onion

1 tablespoon sugar

1. If the artichoke hearts are large, cut them in quarters. If they are small, cut them in half. You should have about 40 pieces.

2. Combine the marinade ingredients in a blender, and process for 30 seconds, or until smooth. Place the artichoke hearts in a shallow dish, and pour the marinade over them. Cover and chill for several hours or overnight.

3. Cut each ham slice into ^{1}/₂-inch strips. Drain the artichoke hearts, and discard the marinade. Wrap a ham strip around each artichoke piece, and secure with a wooden toothpick.

4. Place the wrapped artichokes in a shallow baking dish, and bake at 350°F for 10 to 15 minutes, or until thoroughly heated. Transfer to a serving platter, and serve hot.

NUTRITIONAL FACTS (PER APPETIZER)
Calories: 11   Carbohydrates: 1 g   Cholesterol: 2 mg
Fat: 0.3 g   Fiber: 1 g   Protein: 1.1 g   Sodium: 49 mg

You Save: Calories: 17   Fat: 2 g

BOUNTIFUL BREADS AND MUFFINS

Whole Wheat Banana-Nut Bread

Yield: 16 slices

2 cups whole wheat pastry flour

1/2 cup sugar

1 teaspoon baking powder

1 teaspoon baking soda

1/2 teaspoon ground nutmeg

2 cups mashed very ripe banana (about 4 large)

1/2 cup chopped walnuts

1. Place the flour, sugar, baking powder, baking soda, and nutmeg in a large bowl, and stir to mix well. Add the banana, and stir just until the dry ingredients are moistened. Fold in the walnuts.

2. Coat an 8-x-4-inch loaf pan with nonstick cooking spray. Spread the mixture evenly in the pan, and bake at 325°F for about 55 minutes, or just until a wooden toothpick inserted in the center of the loaf comes out clean.

3. Remove the bread from the oven, and let sit for 10 minutes. Invert the loaf onto a wire rack, turn right side up, and cool to room temperature. Wrap the loaf in aluminum foil or plastic wrap, and let sit overnight before slicing and serving. (Overnight storage will give the loaf a softer, moister crust, and allow the flavors to develop.) Refrigerate any leftovers not eaten within 24 hours.

NUTRITIONAL FACTS (PER SLICE)

Calories: 125   Carbohydrates: 24 g   Cholesterol: 0 mg
Fat: 2.6 g   Fiber: 2.6 g   Protein: 3.3 g   Sodium: 102 mg

You Save: Calories: 94   Fat: 7.5 g

Fresh Pear Bread

Yield: 16 slices

2 cups whole wheat pastry flour

1/2 cup sugar

1 teaspoon baking powder

1 teaspoon baking soda

1/4 teaspoon ground nutmeg

1/4 teaspoon ground cinnamon

3/4 cup pear nectar

1 teaspoon vanilla extract

1 1/3 cups finely chopped peeled pear (about 1 1/2 medium)

1/3 cup dried currants or dark raisins

1. Place the flour, sugar, baking powder, baking soda, nutmeg, and cinnamon in a large bowl, and stir to mix well. Add the nectar, vanilla extract, and pears, and stir just until the dry ingredients are moistened. Fold in the currants or raisins.

2. Coat an 8-x-4-inch loaf pan with nonstick cooking spray. Spread the mixture evenly in the pan, and bake at 325°F for about 45 minutes, or just until a wooden toothpick inserted in the center of the loaf comes out clean.

3. Remove the bread from the oven, and let sit for 10 minutes. Invert the loaf onto a wire rack, turn right side up, and cool to room temperature. Wrap the loaf in aluminum foil or plastic wrap, and let sit overnight before slicing and serving. (Overnight storage will give the loaf a softer, moister crust, and allow the flavors to develop.) Refrigerate any leftovers not eaten within 24 hours.

NUTRITIONAL FACTS (PER SLICE)
Calories: 100   Carbohydrates: 24 g   Cholesterol: 0 mg
Fat: 0.3 g   Fiber: 2.5 g   Protein: 2.2 g   Sodium: 103 mg

You Save: Calories: 80   Fat: 7.4 g

Apricot-Oat Scones

Yield: 12 servings

1²/₃ cups unbleached flour

1 cup quick-cooking oats

2 tablespoons sugar

1 tablespoon baking powder

¹/₄ teaspoon baking soda

3 tablespoons reduced-fat margarine or light butter, cut into pieces

¹/₄ cup fat-free egg substitute, divided

¹/₂ cup nonfat or low-fat buttermilk

¹/₄ cup plus 2 tablespoons chopped dried apricots

1. Place the flour, oats, sugar, baking powder, and baking soda in a medium-sized bowl, and stir to mix well. Using a pastry cutter or 2 knives, cut in the margarine or butter until the mixture resembles coarse crumbs. Stir in 3 tablespoons of the egg substitute and just enough of the buttermilk to form a stiff dough. Stir in the apricots.

2. Form the dough into a ball, and turn onto a lightly floured surface. With floured hands, pat the dough into a 7-inch circle.

3. Coat a baking sheet with nonstick cooking spray. Place the dough on the sheet, and use a sharp knife to cut it into 12 wedges. Pull the wedges out slightly to leave a ¹/₄-inch space between them. Brush the tops lightly with the remaining tablespoon of egg substitute.

4. Bake at 375°F for 16 to 18 minutes, or until lightly browned. Transfer to a serving plate, and serve hot.

NUTRITIONAL FACTS (PER SCONE)

Calories: 123   Carbohydrates: 22.5 g   Cholesterol: 0 mg

Fat: 2 g   Fiber: 1.6 g   Protein: 3.7 g   Sodium: 132 mg

You Save: Calories: 60 Fat: 6.9 g

Fruitful Bran Muffins

For variety, substitute mashed banana or apricot baby food for the applesauce.

Yield: 12 muffins

1 cup wheat bran	1 teaspoon baking soda
1 cup nonfat or low-fat buttermilk	1/4 cup plus 2 tablespoons honey
1/4 cup plus 2 tablespoons unsweetened applesauce	2 egg whites, lightly beaten, or 1/4 cup fat-free egg substitute
1 1/2 cups whole wheat pastry flour or unbleached flour	1/2 cup dark raisins, chopped pitted prunes, or chopped dried apricots

1. Place the bran, buttermilk, and applesauce in a medium-sized bowl. Stir to mix well, and set aside for 15 minutes.

2. Place the flour and baking soda in a large bowl, and stir to mix well. Add the bran mixture, honey, and egg whites or egg substitute, and stir just until the dry ingredients are moistened. Fold in the raisins, prunes, or apricots.

3. Coat muffin cups with nonstick cooking spray, and fill three-fourths full with the batter. Bake at 350°F for about 16 minutes, or just until a wooden toothpick inserted in the center of a muffin comes out clean.

4. Remove the muffin tin from the oven, and allow it to sit for 5 minutes before removing the muffins. Serve warm or at room temperature. Refrigerate any leftovers not eaten within 24 hours.

NUTRITIONAL FACTS (PER MUFFIN)

Calories: 120   Carbohydrates: 24 g   Cholesterol: 0 mg

Fat: 0.7 g   Fiber: 4.3 g   Protein: 4.5 g   Sodium: 145 mg

You Save: Calories: 60 Fat: 7 g

BREAKFASTS FOR CHAMPIONS

Banana Buttermilk Pancakes

Yield: 15 pancakes

1½ cups whole wheat pastry flour

1 tablespoon sugar

1 teaspoon baking soda

1¾ cups nonfat or low-fat buttermilk

¼ cup fat-free egg substitute

1½ cups sliced banana (about 1½ medium)

¼ cup honey-toasted wheat germ

1. Place the flour, sugar, and baking soda in a medium-sized bowl, and stir to mix well. Add the buttermilk and egg substitute, and stir to mix well. Fold in the bananas and wheat germ.

2. Coat a griddle or large skillet with nonstick cooking spray, and preheat over medium heat until a drop of water sizzles when it hits the heated surface. (If using an electric griddle, heat the griddle according to the manufacturer's directions.)

3. For each pancake, pour ¼ cup of batter onto the griddle, and spread into a 4-inch circle. Cook for 1 minute and 30 seconds, or until the top is bubbly and the edges are dry. Turn and cook for an additional minute, or until the second side is golden brown. As the pancakes are done, transfer them to a serving plate and keep warm in a preheated oven.

4. Serve hot, topped with honey or maple syrup.

Variation
To make Banana Buckwheat Pancakes, substitute ¾ cup
of buckwheat flour for ¾ cup of the whole wheat flour.

NUTRITIONAL FACTS (PER PANCAKE)
Calories: 78   Carbohydrates: 14.3 g   Cholesterol: 1 mg
Fat: 0.7 g   Fiber: 1.9 g   Protein: 3.6 g   Sodium: 121 mg

You Save: Calories: 39   Fat: 4.2 g

English Muffin French Toast

Yield: 12 slices

1¹/₂ cups fat-free egg substitute

¹/₄ cup plus 2 tablespoons evaporated skimmed milk

1 teaspoon dried grated orange rind

1 teaspoon vanilla extract

6 whole wheat or oat bran English muffins, split open

1. Place the egg substitute, evaporated milk, orange rind, and vanilla extract in a shallow bowl, and stir to mix well. Dip each muffin half in the egg mixture for several seconds, turning to coat both sides thoroughly.

2. Coat a griddle or large skillet with nonstick cooking spray, and preheat over medium heat until a drop of water sizzles when it hits the heated surface. (If using an electric griddle, heat the griddle according to the manufacturer's directions.)

3. Arrange the English muffin slices on the griddle, and cook for 1¹/₂ to 2 minutes on each side, or until golden brown. As the slices are done, transfer them to a serving plate and keep warm in a preheated oven.

4. Serve hot, topped with honey or maple syrup.

NUTRITIONAL FACTS (PER SLICE)

Calories: 88   Carbohydrates: 15 g   Cholesterol: 0 mg

Fat: 0.5 g   Fiber: 1.5 g   Protein: 5.8 g   Sodium: 191 mg

You Save: Calories: 43   Fat: 4.9 g

Southwestern Omelette

Yield: 1 serving

³/₄ cup fat-free egg substitute

3 tablespoons shredded nonfat Cheddar cheese, or 1 slice nonfat Cheddar cheese

2 tablespoons chopped ham (at least 97% lean)

1 tablespoon chopped green bell pepper

1 tablespoon chopped onion

2 tablespoons chopped tomato or picante sauce

1. Coat an 8-inch nonstick skillet with nonstick cooking spray, and preheat over medium-low heat. Place the egg substitute in the skillet, and let the eggs cook without stirring for about 2 minutes, or until set around the edges.

2. Use a spatula to lift the edges of the omelette, and allow the uncooked egg to flow below the cooked portion. Cook for another minute or 2, or until the eggs are almost set.

3. Arrange first the cheese, and then the ham, peppers, and onions over half of the omelette. Fold the other half over the filling, and cook for another minute or 2, or until the cheese is melted and the eggs are completely set.

4. Slide the omelette onto a plate, top with the tomatoes or picante sauce, and serve immediately.

NUTRITIONAL FACTS (PER SERVING)
Calories: 154   Carbohydrates: 8 g   Cholesterol: 14 mg
Fat: 0.7 g   Fiber: 0.5 g   Protein: 29 g   Sodium: 649 mg

You Save: Calories: 303   Fat: 33.3 g

Potato-Crusted Sausage Quiche

Yield: 5 servings

1 cup fat-free egg substitute

1 cup dry curd or nonfat cottage cheese

1 tablespoon unbleached flour

$1/8$ teaspoon ground black pepper

$1/2$ teaspoon Tabasco pepper sauce

1 cup shredded nonfat or reduced-fat Cheddar cheese

4 ounces smoked sausage or kielbasa (at least 97% lean), diced

2 scallions, finely chopped

2 medium potatoes, scrubbed

1. Place the egg substitute, cottage cheese, flour, pepper, and Tabasco sauce in a large bowl, and stir to mix well. Stir in the cheese, sausage, and scallions. Set aside.

2. Coat a 9-inch deep dish pie pan with nonstick cooking spray. Slice the unpeeled potatoes $1/4$-inch thick, and arrange the slices in a single layer over the bottom and sides of the pan to form a crust. Pour the egg mixture into the crust.

3. Bake uncovered at 375°F for 45 minutes, or until a sharp knife inserted in the center of the quiche comes out clean. Allow to cool at room temperature for 5 minutes before cutting into wedges and serving.

NUTRITIONAL FACTS (PER SERVING)
Calories: 190   Carbohydrates: 24 g   Cholesterol: 16 mg
Fat: 0.7 g   Fiber: 1.8 g   Protein: 22 g   Sodium: 489 mg

You Save: Calories: 304   Fat: 36 g

HOT AND HEARTY SOUPS

Fresh Corn Chowder

Yield: 9 servings

1 cup water

4 cups diced peeled potatoes (about 1 1/2 pounds)

1/2 cup thinly sliced celery

1/2 cup chopped onion

2 1/2 teaspoons chicken bouillon granules

1 1/2 teaspoons dried savory

1/4 teaspoon ground white pepper

4 cups fresh or frozen (thawed) whole kernel corn (about 1 1/2 pounds)

3 cups milk

1/4 cup plus 2 tablespoons instant nonfat dry milk powder

3 tablespoons finely chopped fresh chives or scallions (garnish)

1. Place the water, potatoes, celery, onion, bouillon granules, savory, and pepper in a 3-quart pot, and bring to a boil over high heat. Reduce the heat to low, cover, and simmer for 15 minutes, or until the potatoes are almost tender.

2. Add the corn to the pot. Cover and simmer for 5 minutes, or until the potatoes and corn are tender.

3. Place the milk in a medium-sized bowl, and stir in the milk powder. Add the mixture to the pot, and cook, stirring constantly, for about 5 minutes, or until the mixture is heated through.

4. Remove 4 cups of soup—including both broth and vegetables—from the pot. Place 2 cups of the removed soup in a blender, and place the lid on the blender, leaving the top slightly ajar to allow steam to escape. Carefully process the mixture at low speed until smooth. Return the blended mixture to the pot, and repeat this procedure with the remaining 2 cups of soup.

5. Simmer the soup for 5 additional minutes. Ladle the soup into individual serving bowls, and garnish each serving with a sprinkling of chives or scallions. Serve hot.

NUTRITIONAL FACTS (PER 1-CUP SERVING)
Calories: 164   Carbohydrates: 31 g   Cholesterol: 2 mg
Fat: 1.1 g   Fiber: 3.1 g   Protein: 7.8 g   Sodium: 360 mg

You Save: Calories: 122   Fat: 16 g

Split Pea Soup With Ham

Yield: 6 cups

1¹/₂ cups split peas, sorted

1 can (14¹/₄ ounces) unsalted chicken broth

2¹/₂ cups water

1 medium yellow onion, chopped

1 medium carrot, peeled, halved lengthwise, and sliced

1 stalk celery, thinly sliced (include the leaves)

6 ounces ham (at least 97% lean), diced

1 bay leaf

¹/₄ teaspoon ground black pepper

1. Place the peas in a 3-quart pot, and cover with water. Discard any peas that float to the top. Drain the peas well and return them to the pot.

2. Add all of the remaining ingredients to the pot, and bring to a boil over high heat. Reduce the heat to low, cover, and simmer, stirring occasionally, for about 45 minutes to 1 hour, or until the peas are soft and the liquid is thick.

3. Ladle the soup into individual serving bowls, and serve hot.

NUTRITIONAL FACTS (PER 1-CUP SERVING)
Calories: 211   Carbohydrates: 32.7 g   Cholesterol: 15 mg
Fat: 0.9 g   Fiber: 4.7 g   Protein: 18 g   Sodium: 333 mg

You Save: Calories: 56   Fat: 6.4 g

Pasta Fagioli Soup

Yield: 12 servings

1 pound 95% lean ground beef or ground turkey breast

1 large onion, chopped

1 large carrot, peeled, halved, and sliced

2 large stalks celery, thinly sliced (include the leaves)

2 cans (1 pound each) unsalted tomatoes, crushed

1 teaspoon dried basil

1 teaspoon dried oregano

1 teaspoon crushed fresh garlic

¹/₄ teaspoon ground black pepper

3 cups beef broth

1 can (1 pound) navy or garbanzo beans, rinsed and drained

6 ounces elbow macaroni or ziti pasta

1. Place the ground meat in a 4-quart pot, and brown over medium heat, stirring constantly to crumble, until the meat is no longer pink. Drain off any excess fat. (If the meat is 95-percent lean, there should be no fat.)

2. Add the onion, carrot, celery, tomatoes, seasonings, and beef broth to the pot, and bring to a boil over high heat. Reduce the heat to low, cover, and simmer for 15 minutes, or until the vegetables are tender.

3. Add the beans and pasta to the pot, cover, and simmer for 7 to 9 minutes, or just until the pasta is al dente. (Be careful not to overcook, as the pasta will continue to soften as long as it remains in the hot soup.)

4. Ladle the soup into individual serving bowls, and serve hot.

NUTRITIONAL FACTS (PER 1-CUP SERVING)
Calories: 154   Carbohydrates: 20 g   Cholesterol: 25 mg
Fat: 2.4 g   Fiber: 3.5 g   Protein: 13 g   Sodium: 295 mg

You Save: Calories: 61   Fat: 7 g

Lentil and Sausage Soup

Yield: 9 cups

1 1/2 cups dried brown lentils, sorted

8 ounces smoked sausage or kielbasa (at least 97% lean), sliced 1/4 inch thick

1 cup sliced peeled carrots (about 1 medium)

1 cup diced unpeeled potatoes (about 1 medium)

1 medium yellow onion, chopped

6 cups water

1 1/4 teaspoons instant chicken bouillon granules

2 bay leaves

1/4 teaspoon ground black pepper

2 tablespoons tomato paste

1. Place the lentils in a 4-quart pot, and cover with water. Discard any lentils that float to the top. Drain the lentils well and return them to the pot.

2. Add all of the remaining ingredients except for the tomato paste to the pot, and bring to a boil over high heat. Reduce the heat to low, cover, and simmer for 30 minutes, or until the lentils are soft.

3. Stir in the tomato paste, and simmer for 5 additional minutes. Ladle the soup into individual serving bowls, and serve hot.

NUTRITIONAL FACTS (PER 1-CUP SERVING)
Calories: 163   Carbohydrates: 25.3 g   Cholesterol: 11 mg
Fat: 0.9 g   Fiber: 5.1 g   Protein: 13.4 g   Sodium: 366 mg

You Save: Calories: 108   Fat: 11.4 g

Golden Turkey Noodle Soup

Yield: 8 servings

6¹/₂ cups unsalted chicken broth or water

1¹/₂ cups diced peeled sweet potatoes
(about 1 1/2 medium)

1 medium onion, chopped

2 teaspoons chicken bouillon granules

¹/₈ teaspoon ground white pepper

1 medium carrot, peeled and diced

1 stalk celery, thinly sliced (include
the leaves)

4 ounces medium no-yolk noodles

2 cups diced cooked turkey or
chicken breast

1. Place the broth or water, sweet potatoes, onion, bouillon granules, and pepper in a 3-quart pot, and bring to a boil over high heat. Reduce the heat to low, cover, and simmer for 15 minutes, or until the potatoes are tender.

2. Remove the pot from the heat. Using a slotted spoon, transfer the sweet potatoes to a blender. Add 1¹/₂ cups of the hot broth, and place the lid on the blender, leaving the top slightly ajar to allow steam to escape. Carefully process the mixture at low speed until smooth.

3. Return the blended mixture to the pot, and place over high heat. Add the carrots and celery, and bring the mixture to a boil. Reduce the heat to low, cover, and simmer for 6 to 8 minutes, or until the vegetables are barely tender.

4. Add the noodles and turkey or chicken to the pot, cover, and simmer, stirring occasionally, for about 8 minutes, or just until the noodles are al dente. (Be careful not to overcook, as the pasta will continue to soften as long as it remains in the hot soup.)

5. Ladle the soup into individual serving bowls, and serve hot.

NUTRITIONAL FACTS (PER 1-CUP SERVING)
Calories: 151   Carbohydrates: 23 g   Cholesterol: 30 mg
Fat: 0.9 g   Fiber: 1.7 g   Protein: 13 g   Sodium: 287 mg

You Save: Calories: 55   Fat: 6 g

SENSATIONAL SALADS

Fancy Fruit Salad

Yield: 9 servings

1 can (1 pound) apricot halves in juice, undrained

1 can (8 ounces) crushed pineapple in juice, undrained

1 can (12 ounces) apricot nectar

2 packages (4-serving size) sugar-free or regular orange gelatin mix

1 block (8 ounces) nonfat cream cheese

1. Drain the fruits well, reserving the juice. Cut the apricot halves in half, and set aside along with the drained pineapple. Place the juices and nectar in a 1-quart measuring cup. Add enough water to bring the volume to $3^1/2$ cups. Set aside.

2. Place 1 package of the gelatin in a heatproof medium-sized bowl, and set aside. Place 1 cup of the juice mixture in a small pot, and bring to a boil. Pour the boiling juice over the gelatin mix, and stir to dissolve the gelatin. Add 1 cup of the room temperature juice mixture to the gelatin mixture, and stir to mix well.

3. Chill the gelatin mixture for about 1 hour and 15 minutes, or until it is thick, but not set. Stir in the pineapple and apricots, and pour the mixture into a square 2-quart glass dish. Chill the gelatin for about 1 hour or until it is almost set.

4. Place the remaining package of gelatin mix in a blender. Bring $1/2$ cup of the remaining juice mixture to a boil, and pour over the gelatin. Blend the mixture for about 30 seconds, or until the gelatin is completely dissolved. Add the remaining room temperature juice, and blend to mix well. Add the cream cheese, and blend until the mixture is smooth.

5. Pour the cheese mixture over the fruit mixture in the dish. Chill for at least 6 hours, or until firm. Cut into squares to serve.

NUTRITIONAL FACTS (PER $^3/_4$-CUP SERVING)

Calories: 83   Carbohydrates: 16 g   Cholesterol: 1 mg

Fat: 0.1 g   Fiber: 1 g   Protein: 4.4 g   Sodium: 125 mg

You Save: Calories: 73   Fat: 9.9 g

Company Carrot-Raisin Salad

Yield: 8 servings

5 cups grated carrots (about 2 pounds)

³/4 cup thinly sliced celery

²/3 cup dark raisins

DRESSING

¹/3 cup nonfat or reduced-fat mayonnaise

¹/4 cup frozen apple juice concentrate, thawed

1. Place the carrots, celery, and raisins in a large bowl, and toss to mix well.

2. Place the dressing ingredients in a small bowl, and stir to mix well. Pour the dressing over the carrot mixture, and toss to mix well.

3. Cover the salad, and chill for several hours or overnight before serving.

NUTRITIONAL FACTS (PER ²/3-CUP SERVING)

Calories: 103   Carbohydrates: 23 g   Cholesterol: 0 mg

Fat: 0.3 g   Fiber: 3 g   Protein: 1.5 g   Sodium: 156 mg

You Save: Calories: 163   Fat: 17.8 g

All-American Potato Salad

Yield: 8 servings

2 pounds medium-sized red potatoes, unpeeled

¹/3 cup thinly sliced celery

¹/3 cup finely chopped onion

¹/3 cup grated carrot

2 tablespoons sweet pickle relish

DRESSING

¹/3 cup nonfat or reduced-fat mayonnaise

¹/3 cup nonfat sour cream

2 tablespoons spicy mustard

¹/4 teaspoon ground black pepper

1. Cut the potatoes into ³/4-inch pieces. (There should be 6 cups.) Place in a microwave or stovetop steamer, cover, and cook at high power or over medium-high heat for 8 to 10 minutes, or until tender. Alternatively, place the potatoes in a 3-quart pot, cover with water, and bring to a boil over high heat. Reduce the heat to medium-low, cover, and cook for about 8 minutes, or until tender. Rinse with cool water and drain well.

2. Place the potatoes in a large bowl. Add the celery, onion, carrot, and relish, and toss gently to mix.

3. Place the dressing ingredients in a small bowl, and stir to mix well. Add the dressing to the potato mixture, and toss gently to mix.

4. Cover the salad, and chill for at least 2 hours before serving.

NUTRITIONAL FACTS (PER 3/4-CUP SERVING)
Calories: 140   Carbohydrates: 31 g   Cholesterol: 0 mg
Fat: 0.2 g   Fiber: 2.9 g   Protein: 3.5 g   Sodium: 190 mg

You Save: Calories: 129   Fat: 15.2 g

Pacific Chicken Salad

Yield: 6 servings

3 cups cooked brown rice

2 cups diced cooked chicken or turkey breast (about 10 ounces)

2 cups diced fresh pineapple, or 1 can (20 ounces) unsweetened pineapple chunks, drained

1 can (8 ounces) sliced water chestnuts, drained

3/4 cup celery cut into matchstick-sized pieces

DRESSING

1/2 cup nonfat or reduced-fat mayonnaise

2 tablespoons mango chutney

1 teaspoon curry powder

1/4 teaspoon ground white pepper

1/4 teaspoon ground ginger

1. Place the rice, chicken or turkey, pineapple, water chestnuts, and celery in a large bowl, and toss to mix well.

2. Place the dressing ingredients in a small bowl, and stir to mix well. Pour the dressing over the rice mixture, and toss to mix.

3. Cover the salad, and chill for several hours before serving.

NUTRITIONAL FACTS (PER 1 1/3-CUP SERVING)
Calories: 239   Carbohydrates: 38 g   Cholesterol: 36 mg
Fat: 1.9 g   Fiber: 3.5 g   Protein: 17.4 g   Sodium: 213 mg

You Save: Calories: 152   Fat: 18.4 g

Pasta Salad Niçoise

Yield: 5 servings

8 ounces mostaccioli or other
   tube-shaped pasta

1 1/2 cups young tender fresh green
   beans

1 can (9 ounces) albacore tuna in spring
   water, drained

2 3/4 cups chopped frozen (thawed) or
   canned (drained) artichoke hearts

3/4 cup matchstick-sized pieces of red
   bell pepper

1/2 cup diced red onion

1/3 cup sliced black olives

2 tablespoons finely chopped fresh
   lemon thyme, or 2 teaspoons dried
   thyme

DRESSING

1/2 cup fat-free Italian salad dressing

1 tablespoon Dijon mustard

3/4 teaspoon crushed fresh garlic

1. Cook the pasta until almost al dente according to package directions. About 3 minutes before the pasta is done, add the green beans, and cook until the beans are crisp-tender and the pasta is al dente. Drain well, rinse with cool water, and drain again. Return the pasta and green beans to the pot.

2. Add the tuna, artichoke hearts, red pepper, onion, olives, and thyme to the pasta mixture, and toss gently to mix well.

3. Place the dressing ingredients in a small bowl, and stir to mix well. Pour the dressing over the pasta mixture, and toss gently to mix.

4. Transfer the salad to a serving bowl, cover, and chill for at least 2 hours before serving.

NUTRITIONAL FACTS (PER 1 3/4-CUP SERVING)

Calories: 284   Carbohydrates: 46 g   Cholesterol: 14 mg
Fat: 2.5 g   Fiber: 4.5 g   Protein: 19.6 g   Sodium: 543 mg

You Save: Calories: 149   Fat: 16.9 g

SAVORY SIDE DISHES

Skillet Squash and Onions

Yield: 6 servings

1¹/₂ pounds zucchini or yellow squash (about 4 to 5 medium zucchini or 8 to 10 medium yellow squash)

1 medium yellow onion, sliced ¹/₄-inch thick

2 tablespoons water

2 teaspoons butter-flavored sprinkles

¹/₄ teaspoon ground black pepper

1 tablespoon minced fresh dill, or 1 teaspoon dried

1. Cut each squash in half lengthwise; then cut each half into ¹/₄-inch-thick slices. (There should be about 6 cups of squash. Adjust the amount if necessary.)

2. Place the squash and onions in a large nonstick skillet. Sprinkle the water, butter-flavored sprinkles, pepper, and dill over the top.

3. Place the skillet over medium heat, cover, and cook, stirring occasionally, for 7 to 9 minutes, or just until the vegetables are tender. Serve hot.

NUTRITIONAL FACTS (PER ²/₃-CUP SERVING)
Calories: 25   Carbohydrates: 4.3 g   Cholesterol: 0 mg
Fat: 0.2 g   Fiber: 1.6 g   Protein: 1.5 g   Sodium: 30 mg

You Save: Calories: 45   Fat: 5 g

Crispy Cajun Fries

Yield: 6 servings

1¹/₂ pounds unpeeled baking potatoes (about 3 extra large)

1 egg white, lightly beaten, or 2 tablespoons fat-free egg substitute

Nonstick cooking spray

COATING

1¹/₂ teaspoons ground paprika

1¹/₂ teaspoons Cajun seasoning

1. Place the coating ingredients in a small dish, and stir to mix well. Set aside.

2. Scrub the potatoes, dry well, and cut into ³/₈-inch-thick strips. Place the potatoes in a large bowl. Pour the egg white or egg substitute over the potatoes, and toss to coat evenly. Sprinkle the coating over the potatoes, and toss again to coat.

3. Coat a large baking sheet with nonstick cooking spray, and arrange the potatoes in a single layer on the sheet, making sure that the potato strips are not touching one another.

4. Spray the tops lightly with cooking spray, and bake at 400°F for 15 minutes. Turn the potatoes with a spatula, and bake for 10 to 15 additional minutes, or until nicely browned and tender. Serve hot.

NUTRITIONAL FACTS (PER SERVING)
Calories: 129   Carbohydrates: 28 g   Cholesterol: 0 mg
Fat: 0.3 g   Fiber: 2.7 g   Protein: 3.3 g   Sodium: 98 mg

You Save: Calories: 263   Fat: 21.5 g

Pineapple-Sweet Potato Casserole

Yield: 8 servings

1 can (29 ounces) canned sweet potatoes, drained

1 can (8 ounces) crushed pineapple in juice, undrained

$1/4$ teaspoon ground cinnamon

2 teaspoons butter-flavored sprinkles

$1/4$ cup golden raisins or chopped pecans

1 cup miniature marshmallows

1. Cut the potatoes into bite-sized pieces, and place in a large bowl. Add the pineapple with its juice, cinnamon, butter-flavored sprinkles, and raisins or pecans, and toss to mix well.

2. Coat a 9-inch glass pie pan with nonstick cooking spray, and place the sweet potato mixture in the dish. Top with the marshmallows.

3. Bake at 350°F for about 35 minutes, or until the sweet potato mixture is bubbly and the top is lightly browned. If the top starts to brown too quickly, loosely cover the dish with aluminum foil during the last 10 minutes of baking. Serve hot.

NUTRITIONAL FACTS (PER SERVING)
Calories: 130   Carbohydrates: 31.5 g   Cholesterol: 0 mg
Fat: 0.2 g   Fiber: 3 g   Protein: 1.8 g   Sodium: 54 mg

You Save: Calories: 90   Fat: 12 g

Country-Style Green Beans

Yield: 6 servings

1¹/₂ pounds fresh green beans, cut into 1-inch pieces

1¹/₄ teaspoons instant ham bouillon granules, or 3 ounces ham (at least 97% lean), diced

¹/₂ cup water

1 teaspoon dry mustard

¹/₈ teaspoon ground black pepper

1. Combine the green beans, bouillon granules or ham, water, mustard, and pepper in a 2¹/₂-quart pot, and bring to a boil over medium heat. Reduce the heat to low, and simmer uncovered, stirring occasionally, for 2 to 3 minutes, or until the beans turn bright green.

2. Cover the pot, and simmer, stirring occasionally, for 15 to 20 minutes, or until the beans are tender. Serve hot.

NUTRITIONAL FACTS (PER ²/₃-CUP SERVING)

Calories: 37   Carbohydrates: 6.3 g   Cholesterol: 0 mg
Fat: 0.3 g   Fiber: 3.9 g   Protein: 2.2 g   Sodium: 176 mg

You Save: Calories: 45   Fat: 5 g

Spinach-Noodle Casserole

For variety, substitute frozen chopped broccoli for the spinach.

Yield: 8 servings

5 ounces no-yolk noodles (about 4 cups)

1 package (10 ounces) frozen spinach, thawed and squeezed dry

1 cup nonfat cottage cheese

³/₄ cup shredded nonfat or reduced-fat mozzarella cheese

¹/₂ cup evaporated skimmed milk

¹/₂ cup fat-free egg substitute

¹/₈ teaspoon ground black pepper

TOPPING

2 tablespoons grated Parmesan cheese (use regular, not fat-free)

1 tablespoon Italian-style seasoned bread crumbs

1. Cook the noodles al dente according to package directions. Drain the noodles and return to the pot. Add the spinach, cottage cheese, mozzarella, evaporated milk, egg substitute, and pepper, and toss to mix well.

2. Coat an 8-inch square baking dish with nonstick cooking spray, and spread the noodle mixture evenly in the dish.

3. To make the topping, place the Parmesan and bread crumbs in a small bowl, and stir to mix well. Sprinkle the topping over the noodle mixture.

4. Cover the dish with aluminum foil, and bake at 350°F for 35 minutes. Remove the foil, and bake for 10 additional minutes, or until the dish is heated through and the topping is lightly browned. Remove the dish from the oven, and let sit for 5 minutes before cutting into squares and serving.

NUTRITIONAL FACTS (PER $^3/_4$-CUP SERVING)

Calories: 138   Carbohydrates: 19 g   Cholesterol: 4 mg
Fat: 0.9 g   Fiber: 1 g   Protein: 13 g   Sodium: 288 mg

You Save: Calories: 133   Fat: 18 g

Confetti Corn Pudding

Puréed corn, rather than cream, adds richness to this colorful dish.

Yield: 6 servings

1 pound frozen whole kernel corn, thawed, or 3$^1/_3$ cups fresh, divided

$^1/_3$ cup chopped onion

$^3/_4$ cup plus 2 tablespoons skim milk

$^1/_2$ cup fat-free egg substitute

2 tablespoons unbleached flour

$^1/_4$ teaspoon salt

$^1/_8$ teaspoon ground black pepper

1 tablespoon chopped fresh parsley, or 1 teaspoon dried

$^1/_4$ cup finely chopped green bell pepper

$^1/_4$ cup finely chopped red bell pepper

1. Place 1 cup of the corn and all of the onion, milk, egg substitute, flour, salt, and pepper in a blender or food processor. Process for 1 minute, or until the mixture is smooth. Add the parsley, and process for an additional 10 seconds.

2. Place the corn mixture in a large bowl, and add the remaining corn kernels and the peppers. Stir to mix well.

3. Coat a 1$^1/_2$-quart casserole dish with nonstick cooking spray, and pour the corn mixture into the dish. Bake at 350°F for 1 hour, or until a sharp knife inserted midway between the center of the dish and the rim comes out clean. Remove the dish from the oven, and let sit for 5 minutes before serving.

NUTRITIONAL FACTS (PER 2/3-CUP SERVING)
Calories: 98   Carbohydrates: 18.4 g   Cholesterol: 0 mg
Fat: 0.2 g   Fiber: 2.1 g   Protein: 5.6 g   Sodium: 141 mg

You Save: Calories: 105   Fat: 13 g

PERFECT PASTA DISHES

Slim Spaghetti Carbonara

Yield: 4 servings

8 ounces thin spaghetti

1¼ cups evaporated skimmed milk

¼ cup fat-free egg substitute

⅓ cup nonfat grated Parmesan cheese

¼ teaspoon coarsely ground black pepper

1½ teaspoons crushed fresh garlic

4 slices turkey bacon, cooked, drained, and crumbled

¼ cup thinly sliced scallions

2 tablespoons finely chopped fresh parsley

1. Cook the pasta al dente according to package directions. Drain well, return the pasta to the pot, and cover to keep warm.

2. Place the evaporated milk, egg substitute, Parmesan, and pepper in a small bowl. Stir to mix well, and set aside.

3. Coat a large nonstick skillet with butter-flavored cooking spray, and place the skillet over medium-high heat. Add the garlic, and stir-fry for a few seconds, or just until the garlic begins to turn color and smells fragrant.

4. Reduce the heat under the skillet to medium-low, and add the spaghetti. Slowly pour the milk mixture over the spaghetti, and toss gently for a minute or 2, or until the sauce thickens slightly. Add a little more evaporated milk if the sauce seems too dry.

5. Add the bacon, scallions, and parsley to the skillet mixture, and toss to mix well. Remove the skillet from the heat, and serve hot.

NUTRITIONAL FACTS (PER 1¹/₃-CUP SERVING)
Calories: 339   Carbohydrates: 57 g   Cholesterol: 16 mg
Fat: 3.5 g   Fiber: 1.6 g   Protein: 20 g   Sodium: 428 mg

You Save: Calories: 300   Fat: 36.8 g

Pasta With Crab and Asparagus

Yield: 4 servings

8 ounces penne or sea shell pasta

1/2 pound fresh asparagus spears, cut into 1-inch pieces

6 ounces (about 1 cup) flaked cooked crab meat

1/4 cup grated nonfat or reduced-fat Parmesan

SAUCE

1 cup nonfat ricotta cheese

2 scallions, chopped

2 tablespoons dry sherry

2 tablespoons lemon juice

1/4 teaspoon dried oregano

1/8 teaspoon ground white pepper

1. Place all of the sauce ingredients in a blender or food processor, and process until smooth. Set aside.

2. Cook the pasta until almost al dente according to package directions. Add the asparagus to the cooking water, and cook for another minute, or until the asparagus are crisp-tender. Drain the pasta and asparagus, and return the mixture to the pot.

3. Add the crab meat to the pasta mixture, and top with the sauce. Place the pot over low heat, and, tossing gently, cook until the sauce is heated through. If the sauce seems too dry, add a little skim milk.

4. Serve immediately, topping each serving with a tablespoon of the Parmesan.

NUTRITIONAL FACTS (PER 1 1/2-CUP SERVING)
Calories: 337   Carbohydrates: 51.6 g   Cholesterol: 47 mg
Fat: 1.6 g   Fiber: 2.7 g   Protein: 29 g   Sodium: 232 mg

You Save: Calories: 175   Fat: 24 g

Ragin' Cajun Pasta

Yield: 6 servings

12 ounces fettuccine pasta

1/2 pound cleaned raw shrimp

2 teaspoons crushed fresh garlic

4 ounces smoked sausage or kielbasa (at least 97% lean), thinly sliced

1/2 cup chopped onion

1/2 cup chopped green bell pepper

1 can (14 1/2 ounces) unsalted stewed tomatoes, crushed

1 1/2 teaspoons Cajun seasoning (or more to taste)

1. Cook the pasta al dente according to package directions. Drain well, return the pasta to the pot, and cover to keep warm.

2. While the pasta is cooking, rinse the shrimp with cool water, and pat them dry with paper towels.

3. Coat a large nonstick skillet with olive oil cooking spray, and place over medium-high heat. Add the shrimp, garlic, and sausage, and stir-fry for about 4 minutes, or until the shrimp and sausage are nicely browned.

4. Add the onions and peppers to the shrimp mixture, and stir to combine. Reduce the heat to low, and add the tomatoes, including their juice, and the Cajun seasoning. Cover and simmer for 10 minutes, or until the onions and peppers are tender.

5. Add the pasta to the sauce, and toss gently to mix well. Serve hot.

NUTRITIONAL FACTS (PER 1^2/3-CUP SERVING)

Calories: 299   Carbohydrates: 52 g   Cholesterol: 66 mg

Fat: 2 g   Fiber: 4.8 g   Protein: 18.5 g   Sodium: 320 mg

You Save: Calories: 127   Fat: 16.2 g

Linguine With Clam Sauce

Yield: 4 servings

2 cans (6 ounces each) chopped clams, undrained

8 ounces linguine pasta

1 tablespoon olive oil (optional)

2 teaspoons crushed fresh garlic

1 medium yellow onion, diced

1 cup sliced fresh mushrooms

^{1}/2 cup thinly sliced celery (include the leaves)

1^1/2 teaspoons dried Italian seasoning

1 tablespoon butter-flavored sprinkles

^{1}/8 teaspoon ground white pepper

^{1}/4 cup finely chopped fresh parsley

^{1}/3 cup grated nonfat or reduced-fat Parmesan cheese

1. Drain the clams, reserving ^{1}/2 cup of the juice, and set aside.

2. Cook the pasta al dente according to package directions. Drain well, and return the pasta to the pot. If desired, add the olive oil and toss to mix. Cover the pot and set aside.

3. While the linguine is cooking, coat a large nonstick skillet with nonstick olive oil cooking spray, and preheat over medium heat. Add the garlic, and stir-fry for a few seconds, or until the garlic just begins to turn color and smells fragrant.

4. Add the onions, mushrooms, celery, Italian seasoning, butter-flavored sprinkles, and pepper to the skillet. Add the clams and the reserved juice, and bring to a boil over high heat. Reduce the heat to low, cover, and simmer, stirring occasionally, for 10 minutes, or until the vegetables are tender.

5. Add the cooked linguine and the parsley to the clam mixture, and toss gently until well mixed. Serve immediately, topping each serving with a rounded tablespoon of the Parmesan.

NUTRITIONAL FACTS (PER 1 1/2-CUP SERVING)

Calories: 318   Carbohydrates: 53 g   Cholesterol: 36 mg
Fat: 1.9 g   Fiber: 2.4 g   Protein: 22 g   Sodium: 252 mg

You Save: Calories: 131   Fat: 16.5 g

Lasagna Roll-Ups

*In a hurry? Instead of preparing homemade sauce for your
Lasagna Roll-Ups, use 3 cups of bottled fat-free marinara sauce.*

Yield: 4 servings

8 lasagna noodles

1 cup shredded nonfat or reduced-fat
  mozzarella cheese

FILLING

15 ounces nonfat ricotta cheese

1 package (10 ounces) frozen chopped
  spinach, thawed and squeezed dry

1/2 cup grated carrot

2 tablespoons finely chopped fresh parsley

SAUCE

1 can (14 1/2 ounces) unsalted tomatoes,
  crushed

1 can (6 ounces) unsalted tomato paste

1/4 cup plus 2 tablespoons unsalted
  vegetable broth or water

1 medium yellow onion, chopped

1 teaspoon dried Italian seasoning

1 teaspoon crushed fresh garlic

1. To make the sauce, combine all of the sauce ingredients in a 1 1/2-quart pot, and bring to a boil over medium-high heat. Reduce the heat to low, cover, and simmer for 20 minutes, stirring occasionally.

2. To make the filling, combine all of the filling ingredients in a medium-sized bowl, and stir to mix well. Set aside.

3. Cook the noodles al dente according to package directions. Drain, rinse, and drain again.

4. Coat a 2½-quart casserole dish with nonstick cooking spray. To assemble the roll-ups, arrange the noodles on a flat surface, and spread ⅛ of the filling mixture along the length of each noodle. Roll each noodle up jelly-roll style, and place in the prepared dish, seam side down. Pour the sauce over the roll-ups.

5. Cover the dish with aluminum foil, and bake at 350°F for 30 minutes. Remove the foil, top with the mozzarella, and bake for 10 additional minutes, or until the cheese is melted. Serve hot.

NUTRITIONAL FACTS (PER SERVING)

Calories: 384   Carbohydrates: 58 g   Cholesterol: 22 mg
Fat: 1.4 g   Fiber: 6 g   Protein: 35 g   Sodium: 412 mg

You Save: Calories: 146   Fat: 20 g

HEARTY HOME-STYLE ENTREES

Crispy Oven-Fried Chicken

Yield: 8 servings

8 skinless chicken breast halves with bones (6 ounces each), or 3 pounds combined chicken breast halves, legs, and thighs, skinned

1½ cups nonfat or low-fat buttermilk or plain nonfat yogurt

Nonstick cooking spray

COATING

¾ cup Italian-style seasoned bread crumbs

¾ cup unbleached flour

2 teaspoons ground paprika

1½ teaspoons poultry seasoning, Cajun seasoning, or lemon pepper

1. Rinse the chicken and pat it dry with paper towels. Place the chicken in a shallow nonmetal dish, and pour the buttermilk or yogurt over the chicken. Turn the pieces to coat, cover, and refrigerate for 6 to 24 hours.

2. To make the coating, place all of the coating ingredients in a shallow dish, and stir to mix well. Set aside.

3. Coat a large nonstick baking sheet with nonstick cooking spray, and set aside.

4. Remove one piece of chicken from the buttermilk or yogurt, and roll in the crumb mixture, turning to coat each side well. Lay the chicken on the baking sheet. Repeat with the remaining chicken, arranging the pieces in a single layer.

5. Lightly spray each piece of chicken with the cooking spray, and bake at 400°F for 30 minutes. Carefully turn each piece of chicken with a spatula, taking care that the coating does not stick to the pan. Bake for 20 to 30 additional minutes, or until the meat is tender and the juices run clear when the chicken is pierced. Serve hot.

NUTRITIONAL FACTS (PER SERVING)
Calories: 227   Carbohydrates: 13.6 g   Cholesterol: 83 mg
Fat: 2.3 g   Fiber: 0.3 g   Protein: 35 g   Sodium: 336 mg

You Save: Calories: 169   Fat: 13.5 g

Mexican Skillet Dinner

Yield: 6 servings

1 pound 95% lean ground beef

1 can (1 pound) Mexican-style stewed tomatoes, crushed

2¹/₂ cups fresh or frozen (thawed) whole kernel corn

1 teaspoon crushed fresh garlic

8 ounces whole wheat macaroni

1¹/₃ cups water

1 teaspoon instant beef bouillon granules

1 tablespoon chili powder

¹/₂ teaspoon dried oregano

1. Coat a large, deep skillet with nonstick cooking spray, and preheat over medium heat. Add the meat, and cook, stirring to crumble, until the meat is no longer pink. (There should be no fat to drain off.) Add all of the remaining ingredients, and stir to mix well.

2. Bring the mixture to a boil. Then reduce the heat to low, cover, and simmer, stirring occasionally, for 10 to 12 minutes, or until the pasta is tender and the liquid has been absorbed. If any liquid remains, remove the cover and simmer for several more minutes. Serve hot.

NUTRITIONAL FACTS (PER 1¹/₂-CUP SERVING)
Calories: 311   Carbohydrates: 44 g   Cholesterol: 50 mg
Fat: 4.3 g   Fiber: 6 g   Protein: 24 g   Sodium: 357 mg

You Save: Calories: 102   Fat: 12.7 g

Pot Roast With Sour Cream Gravy

Top round roast—which is sometimes sold as London broil—is one of the leanest cuts available, and can be easily substituted for pot roasts and briskets in any of your favorite recipes.

Excellent

Be sure to cover

Yield: 8 servings

2¹/₂ pounds top round roast or London broil

2 teaspoons crushed fresh garlic

¹/₄ teaspoon coarsely ground black pepper

1 medium yellow onion, thinly sliced

2 bay leaves

³/₄ cup beef broth

1¹/₂ pounds potatoes (about 5 medium), scrubbed and quartered

1¹/₄ pounds carrots (about 6 large), peeled and cut into 2-inch pieces

GRAVY

Meat drippings

1¹/₂ teaspoons instant beef bouillon granules

3 tablespoons unbleached flour

¹/₄ cup water

¹/₂ cup nonfat sour cream

1. Trim any visible fat from the meat. Rinse the meat, and pat it dry with paper towels. Spread the garlic over both sides of the meat, and sprinkle with the pepper.

2. Coat a large ovenproof skillet with nonstick cooking spray, and preheat over medium-high heat. Place the meat in the skillet, and brown for 2 to 3 minutes on each side. Remove the skillet from the heat, and spread the onions over the meat. Place the bay leaves in the skillet, and pour the broth into the bottom of the skillet. Cover tightly, and bake at 325°F for 1 hour and 45 minutes.

3. Remove the skillet from the oven, and carefully remove the cover. (Steam will escape.) Arrange the potatoes and carrots around the meat, cover, and return the skillet to the oven for 45 additional minutes, or until the meat and vegetables are tender. Transfer the meat and vegetables to a serving platter, and cover to keep warm.

4. To make the gravy, discard the bay leaves, and pour the meat drippings into a fat separator cup. Then pour the fat-free drippings into a 2-cup measure. (If the meat was well trimmed, there may not be any fat to remove.) If necessary, add water to the defatted drippings to bring the volume up to 1¹/₄ cups.

5. Pour the drippings mixture into a 1-quart saucepan, add the bouillon granules, and bring to a boil over medium heat. Combine the flour and water in a jar with a tight-fitting lid, and shake until smooth. Slowly pour the flour mixture into the boiling gravy. Cook and stir with a wire whisk until the gravy is thickened and bubbly.

6. Reduce the heat to low, add the sour cream, and whisk just until heated through.

Transfer the gravy to a warmed gravy boat or pitcher, and serve hot with the meat and vegetables.

NUTRITIONAL FACTS (PER SERVING)
Calories: 300 Carbohydrates: 34 g Cholesterol: 59 mg
Fat: 5.2 g Fiber: 4.2 g Protein: 29 g Sodium: 335 mg

You Save: Calories: 165   Fat: 17.5 g

Foil-Baked Flounder

*Baking fish in a foil pouch allows the fish to steam in its own juices,
sealing in flavor and nutrients. Vegetables, wine, and herbs—
not fat or salt—provide added flavor and color.*

Yield: 4 servings

4 flounder, sole, snapper, or orange
  roughy fillets (6 ounces each)

2 teaspoons crushed fresh garlic

2 cups snow peas

2 cups thinly sliced carrots (about 2
  medium)

$^1/_4$ cup chopped scallions

2 tablespoons plus 2 teaspoons minced
  fresh dill

2 teaspoons butter-flavored sprinkles

$^1/_2$ teaspoon ground black pepper

$^1/_4$ cup dry white wine

1. Cut heavy-duty aluminum foil into four 8-x-12-inch pieces, and center a fish fillet on the lower half of each piece. Spread $^1/_2$ teaspoon of garlic over each fillet, and top with $^1/_2$ cup of snow peas, $^1/_2$ cup of carrots, 1 tablespoon of scallions, 2 teaspoons of dill, $^1/_2$ teaspoon of butter sprinkles, $^1/_8$ teaspoon of pepper, and 1 tablespoon of wine.

2. Fold the upper half of the foil over the fish to meet the bottom half. Seal the edges together by making a tight $^1/_2$-inch fold; then fold again to double-seal. Allow space for heat circulation and expansion. Use this technique to seal the remaining sides.

3. Arrange the pouches on a baking pan or directly on the oven rack, and bake at 450°F for about 15 minutes, or until the fish is opaque and the thickest part is easily flaked with a fork. Open each packet by cutting an "X" in the top of the foil, and serve hot.

NUTRITIONAL FACTS (PER SERVING)
Calories: 223   Carbohydrates: 15.5 g   Cholesterol: 82 mg
Fat: 2.3 g   Fiber: 3.2 g   Protein: 35 g   Sodium: 176 mg

You Save: Calories: 100   Fat: 11 g

Lemon-Herb Chicken With Vegetables

Yield: 4 servings

4 boneless skinless chicken breast halves (4 ounces each)

1/4 cup chicken broth

16 medium whole fresh mushrooms (about 8 ounces)

2 medium carrots, peeled, halved lengthwise, and cut into 2-inch pieces

2 medium zucchini, halved lengthwise and cut into 1/2-inch slices

MARINADE

2 tablespoons lemon juice

1 tablespoon brown sugar

1 teaspoon crushed fresh garlic

1/2 teaspoon coarsely ground black pepper

1/4 teaspoon salt

1 teaspoon dried thyme, oregano, or rosemary

1. Rinse the chicken, and pat it dry with paper towels. Place the chicken in a shallow nonmetal container.

2. To make the marinade, place all of the marinade ingredients in a small bowl, and stir to mix well. Pour the mixture over the chicken parts, turn to coat, and cover. Chill for several hours or overnight.

3. Coat a large skillet with nonstick cooking spray, and preheat over medium-high heat. Place the chicken in the skillet, reserving the marinade, and cook for about 2 minutes on each side, or until nicely browned.

4. Reduce the heat to low, and add the reserved marinade, broth, mushrooms, and carrots to the skillet. Cover and simmer for 10 minutes. Add the zucchini, and simmer for 5 additional minutes, or until the chicken is no longer pink inside and the vegetables are tender.

5. Serve hot, accompanying each chicken breast with some of the vegetables and pan juices. Serve over brown rice if desired.

NUTRITIONAL FACTS (PER SERVING)
Calories: 192   Carbohydrates: 14 g   Cholesterol: 72 mg
Fat: 2.3 g   Fiber: 2.7 g   Protein: 29 g   Sodium: 263 mg

You Save: Calories: 120   Fat: 14.1 g

Fiesta Chili

Yield: 8 servings

1 pound ground turkey breast or 95% lean ground beef

1 can (14¹/₂ ounces) unsalted tomatoes, crushed

2 cans (8 ounces each) unsalted tomato sauce

1 can (15 ounces) red kidney beans or black beans, rinsed and drained

1 medium yellow onion, chopped

2 tablespoons chili powder

1¹/₄ teaspoons instant beef bouillon granules

¹/₂ teaspoon ground cumin

1¹/₂ cups fresh or frozen (thawed) whole kernel corn

1 can (4 ounces) chopped green chilies, drained

³/₄ cup shredded nonfat Cheddar cheese

1. Coat a 3-quart pot with nonstick cooking spray, and preheat over medium heat. Add the turkey or beef, and cook, stirring to crumble, until the meat is no longer pink. (There should be no fat to drain off.)

2. Add the tomatoes, tomato sauce, beans, onions, chili powder, bouillon granules, and cumin to the pot, and bring the mixture to a boil. Reduce the heat to low, cover, and simmer for 20 minutes.

3. Add the corn and chilies to the pot. Cover and simmer for 5 minutes, or until the flavors are well blended. Serve hot, topping each serving with a rounded tablespoon of the cheese.

NUTRITIONAL FACTS (PER 1-CUP SERVING)

Calories: 182   Carbohydrates: 19.4 g   Cholesterol: 37 mg

Fat: 2 g   Fiber: 5.4 g   Protein: 21.6 g   Sodium: 369 mg

You Save: Calories: 154   Fat: 15.9 g

MEATLESS MAIN DISHES

Grilled Hummus Pitawiches

Yield: 6 servings

6 whole wheat or oat bran pita pockets (6-inch rounds)

18 fresh spinach leaves

3 medium plum tomatoes, thinly sliced

1 1/2 cups shredded nonfat mozzarella cheese

FILLING

1 can (15 ounces) garbanzo beans, rinsed and drained

1/2 cup sliced scallions

1/4 cup finely chopped fresh parsley

1/4 cup plain nonfat yogurt

1 tablespoon sesame tahini (sesame seed paste)

1 1/2 teaspoons crushed fresh garlic

1/4 teaspoon ground black pepper

1. Place all of the filling ingredients in the bowl of a food processor, and process until smooth. Set aside.

2. Using a sharp knife or scissors, cut each pita round about two-thirds of the way around the edges. Carefully open the pita bread round, and spread 1/4 cup of the filling over the bottom layer. Arrange first 3 spinach leaves, then 3 slices of tomato, and finally 1/4 cup of cheese over the filling.

3. Coat a large nonstick griddle or skillet with nonstick olive oil cooking spray, and preheat over medium heat. Lay the sandwiches on the griddle, and cook for about 2 minutes. Spray the tops of the sandwiches lightly with cooking spray, then flip them over and cook for 2 additional minutes, or until the bread is lightly toasted, the filling is hot, and the cheese is melted.

4. Cut each sandwich into 4 wedges, and serve hot.

NUTRITIONAL FACTS (PER SERVING)

Calories: 293   Carbohydrates: 46 g   Cholesterol: 1 mg
Fat: 4 g   Fiber: 7.4 g   Protein: 18 g   Sodium: 552 mg

You Save: Calories: 121   Fat: 14.6 g

Spring Vegetable Quiche

Yield: 5 servings

1 1/2 cups cooked brown rice

1 egg white

1 cup chopped fresh asparagus or broccoli

1/2 cup fresh or frozen (thawed) whole kernel corn

1/3 cup finely chopped carrots

1/3 cup chopped fresh mushrooms

1/4 cup finely chopped onion

2 tablespoons minced fresh parsley

1 tablespoon unbleached flour

1 cup shredded nonfat or reduced-fat mozzarella cheese

1 cup evaporated skimmed milk

1 cup fat-free egg substitute

2 tablespoons grated nonfat or reduced-fat Parmesan cheese

1. To make the crust, place the brown rice and egg white in a medium-sized bowl, and stir to mix well. Coat a 9-inch deep dish pie pan with nonstick cooking spray, and use the back of a spoon to pat the mixture over the bottom and sides of the pan, forming an even crust.

2. Place all of the remaining ingredients except for the Parmesan in a large bowl. Stir to mix well, and pour into the rice crust. Sprinkle the Parmesan over the top.

3. Bake at 375°F for about 50 minutes, or until the top is golden brown and a sharp knife inserted in the center of the quiche comes out clean. Remove the dish from the oven, and let sit for 5 minutes before slicing and serving.

NUTRITIONAL FACTS (PER SERVING)

Calories: 197   Carbohydrates: 27 g   Cholesterol: 8 mg

Fat: 0.9 g   Fiber: 2.5 g   Protein: 20 g   Sodium: 337 mg

You Save: Calories: 283   Fat: 35.4 g

Fiesta Bean Bake

Yield: 5 servings

1 teaspoon whole cumin seeds

1 medium zucchini, halved and sliced 1/4-inch thick

1/2 cup chopped onion

1/4 cup finely chopped red bell pepper

4 cups cooked brown rice

1 can (15 ounces) pinto or black beans, rinsed and drained

1/2 cup plus 2 tablespoons shredded nonfat or reduced-fat Cheddar cheese

1/2 cup plus 2 tablespoons shredded nonfat or reduced-fat Monterey jack cheese

1. Coat a large nonstick skillet with nonstick cooking spray, and preheat over medium-high heat. Add the cumin seeds, and stir-fry for about 1 minute, or until the seeds smell toasted and fragrant. Add the zucchini, onion, and red pepper, and stir-fry for about 2 minutes, or just until the vegetables are crisp-tender.

2. Remove the skillet from the heat, and toss in the rice and beans. Combine the cheeses in a medium-sized bowl, and toss to mix. Add 1 cup of the cheese to the rice mixture, and toss to mix well.

3. Coat a 2-quart casserole dish with nonstick cooking spray, and spread the rice mixture evenly in the dish. Sprinkle the remaining ¼ cup of cheese over the top, cover with aluminum foil, and bake at 350°F for 30 minutes, or until the casserole is heated through. Remove the foil, and bake for 5 additional minutes, or until the cheese is melted. Serve hot.

NUTRITIONAL FACTS (PER 1¹/₂-CUP SERVING)
Calories: 301   Carbohydrates: 54 g   Cholesterol: 10 mg
Fat: 1.7 g   Fiber: 8 g   Protein: 17.2 g   Sodium: 355 mg

You Save: Calories: 216   Fat: 21.8 g

Curried Lentils

Yield: 5 cups

1 cup dried brown or red lentils, sorted

3 cups unsalted chicken broth or water

1 large yellow onion, chopped

2 medium carrots, peeled, halved, and sliced

2 stalks celery, thinly sliced (include the leaves)

1 large apple, peeled and finely chopped

1 teaspoon crushed fresh garlic

1¹/₂ teaspoons instant vegetable or chicken bouillon granules

2–3 teaspoons curry powder

1. Place the lentils in a 2¹/₂-quart pot, and cover them with water. Discard any lentils that float to the top. Drain the lentils well and return them to the pot.

2. Add all of the remaining ingredients to the pot, and bring to a boil over high heat. Reduce the heat to low, cover, and simmer, stirring occasionally, for about 30 minutes, or until the lentils are soft. (If you're using red lentils, cook the mixture for only about 20 minutes.)

3. Serve hot, ladling each serving over brown rice or couscous, if desired.

NUTRITIONAL FACTS (PER 1-CUP SERVING)
Calories: 181   Carbohydrates: 31.7 g   Cholesterol: 0 mg
Fat: 0.7 g   Fiber: 7.2 g   Protein: 12 g   Sodium: 340 mg

You Save: Calories: 120   Fat: 13.6 g

Spicy Pinto Beans

Yield: 7 cups

2 cups dried pinto beans, sorted

5¹/₂ cups unsalted vegetable broth, chicken broth, or water

1 medium yellow onion, chopped

1 teaspoon crushed fresh garlic

1 tablespoon chopped jalapeño pepper

2 teaspoons instant vegetable, ham, or chicken bouillon granules

1¹/₂ teaspoons ground cumin

2 teaspoons chili powder

2 medium tomatoes, diced

¹/₃ cup chopped fresh cilantro or scallions

1. Place the beans in a 3-quart pot, and cover them with 2 quarts of water. Discard any beans that float to the top. Let the beans soak for at least 4 hours. You can let the beans soak for up to 12 hours if desired, but place them in the refrigerator if you are going to soak them for more than 4 hours. (If you are in a hurry, bring the pot of beans to a boil for 2 minutes, remove from the heat, cover, and let soak for 1 hour.) Drain the beans well and return them to the pot.

2. Add all of the remaining ingredients except for the tomatoes and cilantro to the pot, and bring to a boil over high heat. Reduce the heat to low, cover, and simmer, stirring occasionally, for 1 hour and 30 minutes, or until the beans are tender. Periodically check the pot during cooking, and add a little more broth or water if needed.

3. Add the tomatoes to the bean mixture, and cook for 30 additional minutes. Serve hot, topping each serving with some cilantro or scallions. If desired, serve over brown rice.

NUTRITIONAL FACTS (PER 1-CUP SERVING)
Calories: 184   Carbohydrates: 33 g   Cholesterol: 0 mg
Fat: 0.9 g   Fiber: 12 g   Protein: 11 g   Sodium: 289 mg

You Save: Calories: 89   Fat: 11 g

Baked Macaroni and Cheese

Yield: 6 servings

8 ounces elbow macaroni

2$^1/_2$ cups skim milk, divided

3 tablespoons unbleached flour

2 teaspoons dry mustard

8 ounces nonfat processed Cheddar cheese or reduced-fat Cheddar

cheese (about 2 cups shredded or 1$^1/_2$ cups diced)

2 tablespoons finely ground cracker crumbs

Butter-flavored nonstick cooking spray

1. Cook the macaroni al dente according to package directions. Drain well, and return the macaroni to the pot. Set aside.

2. While the macaroni is cooking, place $^1/_2$ cup of the milk and all of the flour and mustard in a jar with a tight-fitting lid. Shake until smooth, and set aside.

3. Pour the remaining 2 cups of milk into a 2-quart pot, and bring to a boil over medium heat, stirring constantly. Add the flour mixture, and cook, still stirring, for about 1 minute, or until thickened and bubbly. Reduce the heat to medium-low, add the cheese, and stir until the cheese melts.

4. Pour the cheese sauce over the macaroni, and toss to mix well. Coat a 2-quart casserole dish with nonstick cooking spray, and spread the macaroni mixture evenly in the dish. Sprinkle the crumbs over the top, and spray the top with the cooking spray. Bake at 350°F for 30 to 35 minutes, or until bubbly around the edges. Remove the dish from the oven, and let sit for 5 minutes before serving.

NUTRITIONAL FACTS (PER 1-CUP SERVING)

Calories: 259   Carbohydrates: 40.5 g   Cholesterol: 2 mg

Fat: 1.2 g   Fiber: 1.1 g   Protein: 21 g   Sodium: 353 mg

You Save: Calories: 171   Fat: 21.1 g

DELIGHTFUL DESSERTS

Carrot Cake With Cream Cheese Frosting

To make Chocolate Carrot Cake, substitute cocoa powder for $^1/_2$ cup of the flour.

Yield: 16 servings

3 cups unbleached flour

1$^1/_2$ cups sugar

2$^1/_2$ teaspoons baking soda

2 teaspoons ground cinnamon

1$^1/_3$ cups orange or apple juice

$^3/_4$ cup fat-free egg substitute

2 teaspoons vanilla extract

4 cups (packed) grated carrots (about 8 large)

$^1/_2$ cup golden or dark raisins

$^1/_2$ cup chopped walnuts or pecans (optional)

CREAM CHEESE FROSTING

1$^1/_2$ blocks (8 ounces each) nonfat cream cheese, softened to room temperature

$^1/_4$ cup plus 2 tablespoons sugar

1$^1/_2$ teaspoons vanilla extract

1$^1/_2$ cups nonfat or light whipped topping

1. Place the flour, sugar, baking soda, and cinnamon in a large bowl, and stir to mix well. Stir in the juice, egg substitute, and vanilla extract. Fold in the carrots, raisins, and, if desired, the walnuts or pecans.

2. Coat a 9-x-13-inch pan with nonstick cooking spray, and spread the mixture evenly in the pan. Bake at 300°F for 50 to 55 minutes, or just until the top springs back when lightly touched and a wooden toothpick inserted in the center of the cake comes out clean. Cool to room temperature.

3. To make the frosting, place the cream cheese in a large bowl. Add the sugar and vanilla extract, and beat with an electric mixer until smooth. Gently fold in the whipped topping. Spread the frosting over the cooled cake and refrigerate for at least 2 hours before cutting into squares and serving.

NUTRITIONAL FACTS (PER SERVING)

Calories: 246   Carbohydrates: 53 g   Cholesterol: 1 mg

Fat: 0.6 g   Fiber: 1.7 g   Protein: 7.3 g   Sodium: 333 mg

You Save: Calories: 258   Fat: 26.4 g

Lemon Cream Cake

Yield: 16 servings

CAKE

1 box (1 pound 2.25 ounces) lemon cake mix

1 package (4-serving size) instant lemon pudding mix

1 cup nonfat sour cream

1 cup fat-free egg substitute

$^1/_2$ cup water

3 tablespoons lemon juice

GLAZE

$^1/_2$ cup powdered sugar

1$^1/_2$ teaspoons lemon juice

1$^1/_2$ teaspoons nonfat sour cream

1. Place the cake and pudding mixes in a large bowl, and stir to mix well. Add the sour cream, egg substitute, water, and lemon juice, and beat with an electric mixer for about 2 minutes, or until well mixed.

2. Coat a 12-cup bundt pan with nonstick cooking spray, and spread the batter evenly in the pan. Bake at 350°F for 40 to 45 minutes, or just until the top springs back when lightly touched, and a wooden toothpick inserted in the center of the cake comes out clean. Be careful not to overbake.

3. Let the cake cool in the pan for 45 minutes. Then invert onto a serving platter and cool to room temperature.

4. To make the glaze, place the powdered sugar, lemon juice, and sour cream in a small bowl, and stir to mix well. Microwave the glaze at high power for 25 seconds, or until hot and runny. Alternatively, place the glaze in a small pot, and cook and stir over medium heat for about 25 seconds. Drizzle the hot glaze over the cake. Let the cake sit for at least 15 minutes before slicing and serving.

NUTRITIONAL FACTS (PER SERVING)

Calories: 195   Carbohydrates: 39 g   Cholesterol: 0 mg

Fat: 2.6 g   Fiber: 0.7 g   Protein: 3.1 g   Sodium: 288 mg

You Save: Calories: 97   Fat: 12.5 g

Blueberry Swirl Cheesecake

Yield: 10 servings

CRUST

5 large (2¹/₂-x-5-inch) reduced-fat
  graham crackers

1 tablespoon sugar

1 tablespoon fat-free egg substitute

FILLING

2 blocks (8 ounces each) nonfat cream
  cheese, softened to room temperature

15 ounces nonfat ricotta cheese

³/₄ cup sugar

¹/₂ cup fat-free egg substitute

¹/₄ cup plus 2 tablespoons unbleached
  flour

1 tablespoon freshly grated lemon rind,
  or 1 teaspoon dried

2 teaspoons vanilla extract

³/₄ cup canned blueberry pie filling

1. To make the crust, break the crackers into pieces, and place in the bowl of a food processor or blender. Process into fine crumbs. Measure the crumbs. There should be ³/₄ cup. (Adjust the amount if necessary.)

2. Return the crumbs to the food processor or blender, add the sugar, and process for a few seconds to mix. Add the egg substitute, and process until the mixture is moist and crumbly.

3. Coat a 9-inch springform pan with nonstick cooking spray, and use the back of a spoon to press the mixture over the bottom of the pan and ¹/₂-inch up the sides, forming an even crust. (Periodically dip the spoon in sugar, if necessary, to prevent sticking.) Bake at 350°F for 8 minutes, or until the edges feel firm and dry. Set aside to cool.

4. To make the filling, place the cream cheese, ricotta, and sugar in the bowl of a food processor, and process until smooth. Add the egg substitute, flour, lemon rind, and vanilla extract, and process until smooth.

5. Spread half of the cheesecake batter evenly over the crust. Then spoon the blueberry pie filling randomly over the batter. Top with the remaining cheesecake batter, and draw a knife through the batter to produce a marbled effect.

6. Bake at 325°F for 1 hour, or until the center is set. (If you use a dark pan instead of a shiny one, reduce the oven temperature to 300°F.) Turn the oven off, and allow the cake to cool in the oven with the door ajar for 30 minutes.

7. Remove the cake from the oven, and chill for at least 8 hours. Remove the collar of the pan just before slicing and serving.

NUTRITIONAL FACTS (PER SERVING)

Calories: 208   Carbohydrates: 36.6 g   Cholesterol: 10 mg
Fat: 0.6 g   Fiber: 0.6 g   Protein: 14 g   Sodium: 346 mg

You Save: Calories: 311   Fat: 33.8 g

Old-Fashioned Peach Cobbler

Yield: 8 servings

FILLING

$1/4$ cup sugar

2 tablespoons cornstarch

$1/4$ teaspoon ground cinnamon

$1/8$ teaspoon ground nutmeg

$1/2$ cup orange juice

$4^1/2$ cups sliced peeled peaches (about 5 medium), or $4^1/2$ cups frozen (thawed) sliced peaches

TOPPING

$3/4$ cup unbleached flour

$1/3$ cup oat bran

$1/3$ cup sugar

$1^1/2$ teaspoons baking powder

$1/2$ teaspoon baking soda

$3/4$ cup nonfat or low-fat buttermilk

1. To make the filling, place the sugar, cornstarch, cinnamon, and nutmeg in a 2-quart pot, and stir to mix well. Add the orange juice, and stir to mix well. Place the pot over medium heat, and cook, stirring constantly, for 3 to 5 minutes, or until the mixture is thickened and bubbly.

2. Remove the pot from the heat, and stir the peach slices into the glaze, tossing gently to coat. Coat a 2-quart casserole dish with nonstick cooking spray, and spread the peach mixture evenly in the dish.

3. To make the batter topping, place the flour, oat bran, sugar, baking powder, and baking soda in a medium-sized bowl, and stir to mix well. Add the buttermilk, and stir just until well mixed.

4. Spread the batter evenly over the fruit, and bake at 350°F for 35 to 40 minutes, or until the topping is golden brown and the filling is bubbly around the edges. (Loosely cover the dish with aluminum foil during the last 10 minutes of baking if the top starts to brown too quickly.) Remove the dish from the oven, and let stand for at least 10 minutes. Serve warm or at room temperature.

NUTRITIONAL FACTS (PER $3/4$-CUP SERVING)

Calories: 172   Carbohydrates: 38.3 g   Cholesterol: 0 mg

Fat: 0.6 g   Fiber: 2.7 g   Protein: 3.3 g   Sodium: 172 mg

You Save: Calories: 145   Fat: 11 g

Very Strawberry Pie

Yield: 8 servings

CRUST

1 cup barley nugget cereal

1/4 cup finely ground pecans

2 tablespoons light brown sugar

3 tablespoons fat-free egg substitute

FILLING

4 cups halved strawberries

GLAZE

1/4 cup plus 2 tablespoons sugar

1/4 cup cornstarch

1/2 cup frozen (thawed) cran-strawberry juice concentrate, or another strawberry juice concentrate blend

1 cup water

1 1/2 teaspoons unflavored gelatin

1. To make the crust, place the cereal, pecans, and brown sugar in a small bowl, and stir to mix well. Stir in the egg substitute.

2. Coat a 9-inch pie pan with nonstick cooking spray, and use the back of a spoon to press the mixture across the bottom and sides of the pan to form an even crust. Bake at 350°F for 12 to 14 minutes, or until the edges are lightly browned. Set aside to cool.

3. To make the glaze, place the sugar and cornstarch in a 1-quart pot, and mix well. Stir in the juice concentrate and water, and bring to boil over medium heat, stirring constantly with a whisk. Reduce the heat to low, and cook and stir for 1 minute, or until the mixture is thickened and bubbly. Remove from the heat, sprinkle the gelatin over the top, and whisk to mix. Set aside for 20 minutes.

4. Place the berries in a large bowl. Stir the glaze, and pour over the berries, tossing gently to coat.

5. Spread the strawberry mixture over the prepared crust, and chill for several hours, or until the glaze is set. Serve cold.

NUTRITIONAL FACTS (PER SERVING)

Calories: 189   Carbohydrates: 39 g   Cholesterol: 0 mg

Fat: 2.4 g   Fiber: 2.7 g   Protein: 2.8 g   Sodium: 107 mg

You Save: Calories: 133   Fat: 11.1 g

Apple-Raisin Bread Pudding

Yield: 8 servings

6 slices stale multigrain or whole wheat bread

1 1/4 cups chopped peeled apples

1/4 cup dark raisins

1/4 cup plus 2 tablespoons sugar

1/2 teaspoon ground cinnamon

2 cups skim milk

3/4 cup fat-free egg substitute

1 1/2 teaspoons vanilla extract

1. Cut the bread into 1/2-inch cubes, and measure the cubes. There should be 6 cups. (Adjust the amount if necessary.)

2. Place the bread cubes in a large bowl. Add the apples and raisins, and toss to mix. Set aside.

3. Place the sugar and cinnamon in a medium-sized bowl, and stir to mix well. Add the milk, egg substitute, and vanilla extract, and stir to mix well. Pour the milk mixture over the bread cube mixture, and stir gently to mix. Let the mixture sit at room temperature for 10 minutes.

4. Coat a 1 1/2-quart casserole dish with nonstick cooking spray, and pour the bread mixture into the dish. Place the dish in a pan filled with 1 inch of hot water.

5. Bake uncovered at 350°F for about 1 hour and 10 minutes, or until a sharp knife inserted in the center of the dish comes out clean. Allow the pudding to cool at room temperature for at least 20 minutes. Serve warm or at room temperature, refrigerating any leftovers.

NUTRITIONAL FACTS (PER 3/4-CUP SERVING)
Calories: 189   Carbohydrates: 37 g   Cholesterol: 1 mg
Fat: 0.8 g   Fiber: 2.5 g   Protein: 8 g   Sodium: 198 mg

You Save: Calories: 128   Fat: 10.3 g

7. Living Fat-Free Away From Home

Many people find that the art of fat-free living is fairly easy to master in their own homes, where they can control the foods that go into their pantry and, ultimately, their meals. However, take these same people out of their healthy home environments, and things can change dramatically. The challenges of eating out—whether grabbing a fast food meal, eating breakfast at the local diner, or enjoying dinner in a fine restaurant—leave many people feeling helpless. Add to this all the lunches and snacks grabbed at the office, holiday parties and special occasion meals, and those occasional trips by car or plane, and low-fat living may seem like an unreachable goal.

What can you do? Plenty. This chapter presents a wealth of ideas for eating healthfully away from home. Even if you are dining at your favorite Mexican restaurant or Italian trattoria, you'll find that many appealing low-fat options are there for the taking. There are also a number of ways to enjoy light and healthy meals when on the road or in the air. Going to the movies? With a little thought, you'll be able to munch your way through the feature without straying from your low-fat lifestyle. Believe it or not, it's even possible to enjoy a holiday party without blowing your fat budget, or to turn a cocktail party into a satisfying *dinner* party. It's easy—once you know the secrets of living fat-free.

HAVING IT YOUR WAY IN RESTAURANTS

Over half of all Americans eat away from home at least once on any given day. And from fast food chains to fine restaurants, a growing number of establishments are changing their menus to keep up with consumer demand for lower-fat foods. But even if a restaurant doesn't have any special low-fat items, there are plenty of strategies you can use to make sure you get what you want when you dine out. Below, you'll find some general guidelines for choosing foods that will allow you to remain within your fat budget. Following that, you'll find specific tips for ordering from each part of the menu.

Basic Guidelines for Eating Out

Before You Go . . .

☐ Don't go to a restaurant ravenously hungry. Have a small snack an hour or two before you go out to eat. By taking the edge off your appetite, you'll have more control when ordering.

☐ Call ahead to ask about the menu, or review the menu posted on the outside window before going inside. Check to see if special requests, such as broiling without butter, are honored.

When You Get There . . .

☐ If you must wait in the bar for your table, order mineral water, club soda with lime, tomato juice, V-8 vegetable juice, or a wine spritzer (white wine mixed with club soda).

☐ Ask questions about portion sizes and cooking methods so there will be no surprises when the order arrives.

☐ If you are prone to overindulgence and tend to be influenced by others, be the first to order so that the foods chosen by those around you won't tempt you.

☐ Request that sauces, dressings, and margarine or butter be served on the side so that you can control the amount used.

☐ Look for menu items that are steamed, broiled, blackened, grilled, roasted, "en papillote" (steamed in parchment paper), stir-fried, stewed, braised, or served "in their own juice."

☐ Avoid menu items that are marinated in oil, fried, pan-fried, or served in cream, cheese, or butter sauces. Also beware of foods that are described as "flaky," "crispy," "creamy," "au gratin," "battered," or "breaded," as these terms usually indicate the use of high-fat ingredients.

☐ Be creative when ordering. Consider ordering an à la carte meal of an appetizer, soup, and salad, rather than a full-course meal.

☐ If portions are large, consider splitting an entrée, or take half home.

☐ Save your splurges for foods you really want, and feel free to indulge once in a while.

☐ Pick one fat per meal. For instance, if having chicken fajitas, choose between the guacamole and the sour cream. Don't have both.

☐ When you are comfortably full, put your napkin on your plate. This will signal your server to remove the plate from the table, and will prevent you from unconsciously nibbling any remaining food.

☐ If you can't resist dessert, share it with a friend—or with several friends.

Making the Most of the Menu

Each part of the menu presents its own challenges and rewards. Many restaurants, such as Ruby Tuesdays, TGI Fridays, Chili's, Bennigan's, Applebee's, Denny's, The

Olive Garden, Chi Chi's, and Cuco's, offer an excellent selection of low-fat fare that is clearly labeled as such on the menu, making choices easy for the fat-conscious consumer. Some restaurants also provide nutritional information for their lighter menu items. But even restaurants that do not have a specific line of low-fat fare will usually have several menu items that are worth choosing. In addition, with just a little modification, many dishes can be made to suit your low-fat specifications. Let's learn how to spot some of the healthier selections in each part of the menu.

Breakfast

Ordering breakfast is not the challenge it once was. Of course, the best choices of all are, and always have been, fresh fruit, applesauce, low-fat or nonfat yogurt, oatmeal, and whole grain cereals with low-fat milk—selections offered by many restaurants. But even if you prefer heartier fare, you'll still find plenty of good options.

If eggs are your pleasure, you will be happy to know that many restaurants, including Village Inn, Denny's, and Bob Evans, will prepare omelettes, scrambled eggs, and other egg dishes with a fat-free egg substitute. Some restaurants will also prepare your eggs with more whites and less yolks if you ask. If you want a breakfast meat to go along with your omelette, choose Canadian bacon. Though high in sodium, this food is quite lean.

Pancakes with fresh fruit or syrup are still another option, and some restaurants even offer whole grain or buckwheat cakes and reduced-calorie syrup. If your restaurant will make French toast with a fat-free egg substitute, this would be another good choice. What about waffles? Most restaurants feature Belgian waffles or dessert-type waffles rather than the waffles you are likely to make at home, which are nutritionally similar to pancakes. Between the milk, eggs, and butter in the Belgian waffle batter—not to mention the butter and whipped cream that come on top—restaurant waffles can be very high in fat, and are best avoided unless the menu specifically states that they are low in fat. To keep the fat in your pancakes and French toast to a minimum, be sure to omit the butter or margarine that is typically spread on top. These items will probably already contain close to 10 grams of fat per serving just from the oil added to the pancake batter plus the fat used on the griddle for cooking.

Best bets for breakfast breads include whole wheat or rye toast, English muffins, and bagels. Be sure to order your toast dry, since restaurants tend to slather on the butter or margarine quite heavily. If you want a spread, jam is a better choice than either butter or margarine. As for side dishes, in the South, grits are a low-fat choice, provided they are served unbuttered. Like white bread, though, grits are a refined food and are low in fiber. Hash brown potatoes will usually come with the equivalent of about 2 teaspoons of fat per serving.

What about breakfast buffets? Avoid them—unless they include a good selection of cereals, fruits, yogurt, and bagels. Between the sausage, bacon, biscuits, gravy, eggs, fried potatoes, and other artery-clogging selections, you can get a whole day's worth of fat and calories from just one trip to the average buffet.

Just how do different breakfast choices compare to one another nutritionally?

The following table lists the calorie and fat contents of some typical restaurant breakfast foods.

Calories and Fat in Selected Breakfast Foods

Breakfast Item	Amount	Calories	Fat
Bacon	2 slices	73	6.2 g
Biscuit, no margarine	2 ounces	221	10.6 g
Canadian bacon	2 ounces	66	3 g
French toast made with whole eggs, plain	3 pieces	452	22g
Grits, unbuttered	1 cup	146	0.5 g
Hash browns	1 cup	220	11 g
Pancakes, no margarine	4 cakes	245	10.5 g
Poached egg	1 egg	75	5 g
Sausage gravy	1/2 cup	206	15.3 g
Sausage links	2 ounces	209	17.7 g
Scrambled egg substitute, cooked in margarine	1/2 cup	99	5 g
Scrambled eggs, cooked in margarine	2 eggs	202	14.8 g
Syrup	1/4 cup	225	0 g
Syrup, reduced-calorie	1/4 cup	115	0 g
Toast, no margarine	2 slices	130	2 g
Toast, with margarine	2 slices	220	12 g
Waffle, Belgian, plain	1 large	529	32.6 g
Waffle, plain	1 large	245	12.6 g

Appetizers

First, consider whether you really want an appetizer. By the time you have an appetizer, salad, bread, and entrée, you may feel uncomfortably full. If you do choose to order an appetizer, try steamed seafood with cocktail sauce, grilled vegetables, or a cup of broth-based vegetable or bean soup. Most other appetizers—fried potato skins topped with cheese and sour cream, fried cheese sticks, fried onion blossoms, cheese-topped nachos, and fried chicken wings served with blue cheese dressing, for instance—will blow your fat budget for the entire day.

Salads

Everyone knows that salads are healthful—low in fat and calories, and high in nutrients and fiber. Beware, though. A low-fat salad quickly becomes a nutritional disaster when high-fat cheeses, meats, and mayonnaise or oil-based dressings are piled on top. People who, with perfectly good intentions, order a grilled chicken Caesar salad, chef salad, or taco salad, are often astounded to learn that they ate an entire day's worth of fat in what they thought was a healthy meal. What can you do to prevent surprises like these? Use the following guidelines to make sure you get the low-fat dish you want.

☐ Order a low-fat or nonfat dressing. Or get the dressing on the side so you can control the amount added to your salad.

☐ When ordering a main dish salad or side salad, inquire about the ingredients, and ask the chef to leave off or limit the high-fat toppings. For instance, if a salad comes topped with shredded cheese, bacon bits, and fried croutons, choose just *one* of these and leave off the rest.

☐ If your salad comes topped with chicken or tuna, check to see that you will be getting pieces of roasted or grilled chicken or tuna, or chunks of water-packed canned tuna—not mayonnaise-dressed chicken or tuna salad.

☐ If your salad comes served in an "edible" bowl made from a deep-fried flour tortilla, request that the salad be served in a regular bowl, and save yourself about 30 grams of fat!

What about the typical salad bar lunch? A pile of fresh crisp greens makes for a good start. But then comes the shredded cheese, hard boiled eggs, fried croutons, and mayonnaise-laden potato or tuna salad, not to mention the dressing. A typical salad dressing ladle holds 2 tablespoons of dressing. For most dressings, this amounts to about 140 calories and 16 grams of fat! All things considered, it would be easy to walk away with over 50 grams of fat on your plate.

Here's a better idea. Start with lettuce or fresh spinach and plenty of fresh vegetables such as tomatoes, carrots, mushrooms, and green peppers. For protein, add some cottage cheese, kidney beans, or garbanzo beans instead of fatty meats and shredded cheeses. Top off your salad with a sprinkling of raisins, if you like. Then keep your salad low in fat by choosing a nonfat or reduced-fat salad dressing. When your salad is this healthy, you can also afford to add a few chopped olives or sunflower seeds. Avoid the mayonnaise-dressed salads like macaroni salad, potato salad, and cole slaw, as well as oil-drenched marinated vegetables. For dessert, select an assortment of fresh fruits. The following table presents nutrition information for some common salad bar ingredients.

Calories and Fat in Selected Salad Bar Ingredients

Salad Bar Item	Amount	Calories	Fat
Bacon bits	1 tablespoon	25	1.5 g
Broccoli	1/2 cup	12	0.1 g
Cantaloupe, diced	1 cup	56	0.4 g
Carrots, grated	1/4 cup	12	0.1 g
Cheddar cheese, shredded	2 tablespoons	57	4.7 g
Cottage cheese (1% fat)	1/2 cup	82	1.2 g
Eggs, chopped	2 tablespoons	26	1.8 g
Fried noodles/croutons	2 tablespoons	29	1.7 g
Garbanzo beans	1/2 cup	100	1.7 g
Ham, diced (87% lean)	1/2 cup	135	9 g
Kidney beans	1/2 cup	108	0.4 g
Lettuce	2 cups	18	0.2 g
Mushrooms, sliced	1/4 cup	5	0.1 g
Olives, sliced	1 tablespoon	10	0.9 g
Parmesan cheese	1 tablespoon	28	1.8 g
Pineapple, crushed	1/2 cup	75	0.1 g
Potato salad	1/2 cup	178	10.3 g
Raisins	1 tablespoon	30	0 g
Strawberries	1 cup	43	0.5 g
Sunflower seeds	1 tablespoon	50	4.5 g
Tomatoes	1/2 cup	19	0.3 g
Tuna salad	1/2 cup	191	9.5 g
Turkey, diced (95% lean)	1/2 cup	90	3.6 g
Blue cheese dressing	2 tablespoons	154	16 g
Italian dressing	2 tablespoons	140	16.4 g
Italian dressing, fat-free	2 tablespoons	30	0 g
Ranch dressing	2 tablespoons	108	11.3 g
Ranch dressing, fat free	2 tablespoons	35	0 g
Oil	1 tablespoon	120	13.6 g
Vinegar	1 tablespoon	2	0 g

Sandwiches

Made properly, a sandwich can be the perfect meal. You get complex carbohydrates and fiber in the whole grain bread or bun; you get protein in the lean filling; and, if your sandwich is piled high enough with lettuce, tomatoes, and other garden-fresh fixings, you get a complete serving of vegetables. At its worst, though, a sandwich is a nutritional nightmare. Take the Ruben, for instance. Six ounces of fatty corned beef topped with a couple of ounces of full-fat cheese and a couple of tablespoons of thousand island dressing can add up to more than 900 calories and 50 grams of fat!

Just about any sandwich shop offers turkey breast or grilled chicken, which will be among the leanest choices available. Another excellent choice is a grilled or blackened fish sandwich, which is featured in many restaurants. Lean roast beef, ham, and turkey pastrami are still other low-fat choices. Many sandwich shops do go overboard on the meat, stuffing in up to 5 ounces—an entire day's meat allotment in a healthy diet. And "overstuffed," "jumbo," "foot long," or "New York-style" sandwiches can be even worse. Inquire about the amount of meat in the sandwich, and, if it is excessive, ask for less meat. Then pile on extra vegetables.

What about cheese? Unfortunately, few sandwich shops offer low-fat cheese, so this ingredient is best left off. As for spreads, be sure to leave off the mayonnaise unless your restaurant offers reduced-fat or nonfat types. If low-fat mayo is not available, choose mustard instead, or try spreading your sandwich with fat-free ranch, Italian, or honey mustard dressing. Many restaurants do have these ingredients on hand for salads, and will be happy to accommodate you.

Where do chicken, tuna, and egg salad fit in? Though many people think of these fillings as "diet food," they're far from it. You'll rarely find these sandwiches made with low-fat or nonfat mayonnaise. And a chicken or tuna salad sandwich made with regular mayo can provide over 500 calories and 30 grams of fat. Vegetarian sandwiches can also supply a surprising amount of fat. The reason? Several ounces of full-fat cheese replace the meat in these creations. A vegetarian sandwich made with 3 ounces of cheese and a tablespoon of mayonnaise will contain close to 600 calories and 40 grams of fat. If you do order a vegetarian sandwich, ask for only 1 ounce of cheese, and hold the mayo. Falafel—deep-fried chickpea patties in pita bread—is another vegetarian sandwich that provides a lot more fat than most people realize. Just 3 ounces of falafel in a pita pocket topped with dressing can deliver close to 500 calories and 25 grams of fat.

Beware of hidden fats in sandwiches. For instance, when ordering a sandwich that comes on a toasted bun, the buns are often first coated with butter or margarine, which can add as much as 10 grams of fat to your sandwich. Submarine sandwiches are usually doused with a liberal amount of oil. With over 13 grams of fat per tablespoon of oil, it pays to make sure that the oil is omitted. Opt for a splash of vinegar or fat-free Italian salad dressing instead.

Side Dishes

Baked potatoes are always a good side dish choice—when the toppings are chosen wisely. To reduce the fat, you can omit the butter and use only the sour cream, which is lower in fat. Even better, try topping your potato with ingredients from the salad bar, such as low-fat ranch dressing or cottage cheese. Salsa makes a tasty fat-free topping, as well. Or bring your own butter-flavored sprinkles to the restaurant.

Another low-fat accompaniment is rice pilaf. Most restaurants also have at least one vegetable of the day that can often be ordered steamed or cooked without fat. If you choose a dish that automatically comes with French fries, don't be afraid to ask for a substitution. Many times, your restaurant will be happy to offer a side order of steamed vegetables, a salad, or a baked potato—though some restaurants will charge extra for the substitution.

Entrées

Look for baked, broiled, grilled, blackened, poached, steamed, or roasted entrées, and choose fish, shellfish, or skinless chicken for the least fat. To prevent surprises, request that little or no fat be added during cooking, and ask that sauces be served on the side. Baked, broiled, blackened, and poached entrées are sometimes served swimming in butter or drenched in creamy sauces. Also look for entrées that don't include excessively large portions of meat. Stir-fries and shish kabobs are often the best choices. If you order a steak, choose a small filet mignon, London broil, or sirloin instead of a large porterhouse or prime rib.

Beware of the classic "dieter's" plate that some restaurants continue to feature. This plate, which typically includes a ground beef patty, a scoop of cottage cheese, and a small salad, easily provides 700 calories, with over half the calories coming from fat! Also beware of foods that are described as being cooked in "cholesterol-free" oil. *All* vegetable oils are cholesterol-free, but they are still pure fat and loaded with calories. One other item to be wary of is the vegetarian special. Although vegetarian meals are meatless, they may include large amounts of fat from nuts, seeds, oil, eggs, and full-fat dairy products. It pays to ask questions.

Desserts

Dessert does not always have to be forbidden. Sorbets, granitas, fruit ices, and poached fruits have always been a good choice. Many restaurants also serve low-fat or nonfat frozen yogurt, which is another good choice. If you opt for something decadent, share it with a friend—or with several friends. After a full meal, just a couple of bites is usually enough to satisfy. A gourmet coffee or cappuccino made with low-fat milk is still another guilt-free way to end a meal.

Many restaurants are now featuring fat-free and "light" desserts. But beware; fat-free does not mean calorie-free, and light may not be as light as you think. For instance, a fat-free fudge brownie topped with nonfat frozen yogurt and fat-free fudge sauce can contain up to 500 calories. And a piece of "light" cheesecake can contain well over 400 calories and 20 grams of fat. Light products by definition must have a third less calories or no more than half the fat of the regular version. If the original version is loaded with fat and calories, the light version can still be quite high in both. Always check to see if nutrition information is given so that you can make an informed decision.

The Joys of Ethnic Cuisine

Ethnic restaurants present a wide range of delicious possibilities for the discriminating diner who is looking for a change of pace. And while specialties like fettuccine

Alfredo are among the highest-fat dishes in the world, dishes like Tandoori chicken are flavored with savory herbs and spices instead of large amounts of fat. If you haven't experimented much with international cuisine, now is a good time to start. You will discover a whole new world of flavors that will greatly expand your dining pleasures. Here are some guidelines for finding the healthiest selections in a wide variety of restaurants.

Chinese Cuisine

Authentic Chinese food is quite low in fat, with small amounts of meat, seafood, or poultry stir-fried with plenty of vegetables and flavorful sauces, and served atop a mound of steamed rice. Unfortunately, American-style Chinese food tends to be a heavier, fattier version of the traditional cuisine. Here are some tips for eating light in your favorite Chinese restaurant.

Foods to Choose

☐ Broth-based soups, like wonton, hot and sour, and egg drop; steamed dumplings.

☐ Stir-fried combinations of seafood, poultry, lean meat, tofu, and vegetables. (Ask for less oil than usual, and no MSG.)

☐ Chop suey; chow mein. (Ask that they be served with rice or unfried noodles instead of fried chow mein noodles.)

☐ Stir-fried noodle dishes, like seafood, chicken, or vegetable lo mein. (Ask for less oil than usual, and no MSG.)

☐ Steamed fish and vegetable dishes.

☐ Steamed rice.

☐ Plum sauce, black bean sauce, sweet and sour dipping sauce, hot mustard sauce, hoisin sauce.

☐ Fortune cookies and fresh fruit.

Foods to Avoid

☐ Fried egg rolls; fried wontons; fried noodles; spare ribs; chicken wings.

☐ Stir-fried dishes that contain battered and deep-fried meats, like sweet and sour pork and lemon chicken.

☐ Entrées made with large amounts of nuts, like cashew chicken.

☐ Dishes made with duck. (Duck is very fatty.)

☐ Egg foo yung.

☐ Crispy fish and crispy chicken. (These dishes are fried.)

☐ Fried rice.

French Cuisine

This cuisine, which features ingredients like eggs, butter, cheese, and creamy sauces, can be a difficult one for the low-fat diner. And French dishes that many people think of as being lighter choices—such as soufflés, quiches, and crêpes—are typically loaded with fat. Nonetheless, if you know what to look for, you can treat yourself to authentic French cuisine without the guilt.

Foods to Choose

☐ Consommé and broth-based soups; steamed mussels.

☐ Broiled, steamed, or poached seafood and poultry. (Order sauces to be served on the side, and ask if butter or oil is added.)

☐ Seafood and poultry cooked en papillote (steamed in parchment paper).

☐ Chicken or fish Provençal (with tomato sauce); chicken or fish cooked with tomato-wine sauce. (Request that as little oil or butter as possible be used to prepare the dish.)

☐ Seafood or vegetable stews, such as bouillabaisse and ratatouille.

☐ Chicken, beef, and veal stews with wine or tomato sauce.

☐ Steamed vegetables; salads with dressing on the side.

☐ French bread without butter.

☐ Sherbets; sorbets; poached fruits; fresh fruits with liqueur.

Foods to Avoid

☐ Vichyssoise (creamy potato soup) and other cream soups; paté (liver, meat, or chicken spreads made with cream, butter, and eggs).

☐ Anything topped with a high-fat sauce, such as hollandaise or béarnaise. (Made with egg yolks and butter, these sauces contain about 200 calories and 20 fat grams per $1/4$ cup.)

☐ Rémoulade sauce (a mayonnaise-based sauce typically served with seafood).

☐ Quiches; soufflés; crêpes. (These dishes are typically made with unhealthy amounts of cream, cheese, butter, and egg yolks.)

☐ Vegetables in cream or butter sauce; salads with oily dressings.

☐ Croissants.

☐ Foods served with crème fraîche (thickened, cultured heavy cream).

☐ Brie, Camembert, Roquefort, Boursin, and other high-fat cheeses.

☐ French pastries and cakes; cheesecake; mousse; Crème Brulée.

Greek Cuisine

Roasted lamb and chicken flavored with lemon, yogurt, and herbs are some of the better selections found on a Greek menu. On the other hand, buttery phyllo-crusted pies, piles of feta cheese, and pools of olive oil can add an unhealthy amount of fat to your meals. The trick is to choose the healthier dishes from this deliciously spicy cuisine.

Foods to Choose

☐ Bean and lentil soups; avgolemono (lemon and egg) soup; vegetable soups; fish soups.

☐ Shish kabobs of roasted lamb or chicken and vegetables.

☐ Baked fish dishes, such as Plaki (fish baked with tomatoes, onions, and garlic) and fish baked in grape leaves; baked chicken dishes. (Request that as little oil or butter as possible be used to prepare the dish.)

☐ Gyro sandwiches.

☐ Orzo (rice-shaped pasta); rice pilafs; bulgur wheat; pita bread.

☐ Fruit compotes; marinated fruits.

Foods to Avoid

☐ Buttery, phyllo-crusted dishes, such as Spanakopita.

☐ Greek salads made with excessive amounts of feta cheese and olive oil.

☐ Dishes topped with creamy or cheesy sauces, like pastitso and moussaka.

☐ Baklava (phyllo pastry layered with butter, nuts, and honey); nut cakes; butter cookies.

Indian Cuisine

Here's a cuisine with plenty to offer the low-fat diner. Healthful legumes, chicken, fish, vegetables, steamed rice, and yogurt are featured throughout the menu. Curry, cumin, coriander, and other flavorful seasonings add exotic flair. But keep in mind that Indian cooks use clarifed butter (ghee) or vegetable oil to prepare dishes like curries, Vindaloos, and rice dishes, and that some chefs have a heavier hand with the fat than others. Always request that your food be prepared with as little butter or oil as possible.

Foods to Choose

☐ Vegetable and dal (lentil or bean) soups.

☐ Chapati (a whole wheat tortilla-like bread); roti and naan (oven-baked flatbreads).

☐ Raita (a cold side dish made of cucumbers or other vegetables with yogurt sauce).

☐ Chutney (a spicy accompaniment to meals).

☐ Vegetable, chicken, or seafood biryanis (rice-based dishes).

☐ Vegetable, seafood, and chicken curry dishes (except for those made with large amounts of coconut or coconut milk).

☐ Chicken or Shrimp Vindaloo (in a hot and spicy tomato, onion, and curry sauce).

☐ Tandoori chicken or fish (chicken marinated in yogurt and spices and baked in a clay oven).

☐ Lamb or chicken kabobs.

☐ Dals (legume dishes).

Foods to Avoid

☐ Coconut soup.

☐ Puri (fried bread).

☐ Samosa (fried turnovers); pakora (fried chicken or vegetable fritters); papadum (crisp fried lentil wafers).

☐ Dishes served with large amounts of nuts or peanut sauce.

☐ Dishes made with coconut milk or cream.

☐ Dishes made with large amounts of ghee (clarified butter).

Italian Cuisine

While Italian menus feature some real fat-budget busters, they also include many truly healthful selections. How can you steer clear of the fat traps? Simply avoid cheese-laden, creamy, and oily dishes, and instead choose the pasta, tomato sauces, vegetables, beans, and breads. Many Italian restaurants offer pasta dishes in half portions. An excellent strategy for ordering a slimming but satisfying dinner is to combine a half-portion of pasta with a soup and salad.

Foods to Choose

☐ Vegetable or bean based soups, like minestrone and pasta fagioli.

☐ Steamed clams or mussels.

☐ Pasta with tomato-based sauces, like marinara, puttanesca, and arrabbiata; pasta with tomato-seafood sauces, like red clam sauce.

☐ Broiled or grilled chicken and fish dishes. (Request that as little oil or butter as possible be used to prepare the dish.)

☐ Chicken cacciatore; chicken or veal piccata or Marsala. (Request that as little oil or butter as possible be used to prepare the dish.)

☐ Seafood stews like Cioppino.

☐ Thin crust pizza with vegetable toppings. (Ask for less cheese and no olive oil splash.)

☐ Baked or broiled polenta with tomato sauce; gnocchi with tomato sauce.

☐ Italian bread; focaccia; bread sticks.

☐ Granita; poached fruits; biscotti; amaretti cookies; cappuccino made with low-fat milk.

Foods to Avoid

☐ Meat and cheese antipasto platters.

☐ Fried calamari and fried mozzarella.

☐ Vegetables marinated in large amounts of olive oil.

☐ Pasta with creamy sauces, like Alfredo and carbonara.

☐ Cheese-laden dishes, like lasagna, cheese manicotti, and cannelloni.

☐ Dishes like eggplant Parmesan and veal Parmesan, which are battered, pan-fried, and covered with cheese.

☐ Dishes made with Italian sausage.

☐ Oily pesto dishes.

☐ Pizza with extra cheese, olive oil, and meat toppings.

☐ Garlic bread.

☐ Cheesecake; tiramisu; Italian pastries and cookies; spumoni; mousse.

Japanese Cuisine

Most Japanese dishes are deliciously low in fat. Grilled or stir-fried chicken, seafood, and lean beef served with vegetables and rice are featured fare. Raw fish served either as sushi or sashimi is also a Japanese favorite. Teriyaki sauce and ginger are frequently used to add savory flavor to dishes.

Foods to Choose

☐ Miso soup; broth-based soups.

☐ Steamed dumplings.

☐ Sushi (vinegared rice, raw fish, and/or vegetables rolled or pressed together into small morsels); sashimi (raw slivered fish, usually served with a dipping sauce).

☐ Yakitori (broiled chicken kabobs); teriyaki dishes; "yakimono" (grilled) dishes; sukiyaki (thinly sliced beef and vegetables in a piquant, slightly sweet sauce).

☐ Stir-fried seafood, chicken, lean beef, or tofu and vegetable combinations.

☐ Udon (wheat) noodles; soba (buckwheat) noodles; rice noodles; steamed rice.

☐ Fried dumplings.

☐ Tempura (batter coated and fried foods).

☐ Tonkatsu (deep-fried pork); torikatsu (deep-fried chicken); katsudon (deep-fried pork, onion, and egg).

☐ Fried rice.

Mexican Cuisine

From fajitas, quesadillas, soft tacos, and burritos garnished with fat-free sour cream and low-fat cheese, to flavorful grilled chicken and fish served with low-fat rice and fresh fruit, many Mexican restaurants now offer a variety of lighter menu items. Some restaurants even have whole wheat tortillas. Beware, though, as traditional Mexican food can be very fatty, and foods cooked with lard or laden with full-fat cheese and sour cream still dominate the Mexican menu.

Foods to Choose

☐ Black bean soup; ceviche (lime marinated seafood salad); gazpacho (chilled tomato and cucumber soup).

☐ Grilled fish and chicken dishes.

☐ Chicken soft tacos; burritos (limit the cheese and sour cream toppings); chicken and vegetable quesadillas (limit the cheese and sour cream toppings).

☐ Chicken, shrimp, and vegetable fajitas. (Ask that they be cooked in little or no oil, and limit the sour cream, guacamole, and cheese.)

☐ Salsa; tomatillo sauce; verde (green) sauce; pico de gallo (tomatoes with onions and hot peppers).

Foods to Avoid

☐ Fried tortilla chips; nachos.

☐ Sour cream; cheese; guacamole.

☐ Fried entrées like chimichangas and chili rellenos.

☐ Enchiladas (the tortillas are typically softened by drenching in oil).

☐ Refried beans and Mexican rice side dishes. (Both usually contain an unhealthy amount of lard or other fat.)

Thai Cuisine

This flavorful cuisine has much to offer the discriminating diner. Thai dishes typically combine small amounts of meats, seafood, chicken, or tofu with lots of vegetables, noodles, rice, and spicy curry, chili, and fish sauces. Lime juice, lemon grass, and basil also add flavor to this exotic fare.

Foods to Choose

☐ Broth-based soups, like Tom Yum Gai (chicken with vegetables and Thai seasonings) and Tom Yum Goong (shrimp with vegetables and Thai seasonings); steamed dumplings.

☐ Stir-fried combinations of seafood, chicken, tofu, lean meat, and vegetables. (Request that as little oil as possible be used to prepare the dish.)

☐ Sweet and sour dishes. (The meat is not battered and deep-fried like the Chinese versions.)

☐ Pad Jaa and other stir-fried noodle dishes made with vegetables and seafood, chicken, tofu, or lean meat. (Request that as little oil as possible be used to prepare the dish.)

☐ Dishes made with basil sauce, lime sauce, chili sauce, and fish sauce.

Foods to Avoid

☐ Coconut soup, chicken wings, egg rolls, wontons, and other fried appetizers.

☐ Dishes made with duck. (Duck is very fatty.)

☐ Deep-fried dishes, like crispy noodles and crispy fish.

☐ Fried rice dishes.

☐ Fried noodles.

☐ Dishes made with coconut milk.

☐ Dishes made with large amounts of nuts, peanuts, or peanut sauce.

A Word About Buffets and Food Bars

These types of restaurants invite overeating. The combination of a bounty of foods with an all-you-can-eat-for-a-single-price tag, spells disaster for many people. Even if you sample just a little of everything, you can walk away with over 1,000 calories on your plate. And these places definitely don't specialize in healthy food.

If you feel your resolve slip when examining the unlimited choices on a buffet table, consider avoiding those restaurants that feature them. If you do choose to eat at a buffet, peruse the table thoroughly before putting any food on your plate. Concentrate on filling your plate with the most nutritious selections. Then, if you like, indulge in a small portion of something decadent.

Fast Foods With Less Fat

Chosen wisely, even fast foods can fit into a low-fat diet. The biggest boon to the fast food menu has been grilled chicken. Salads with low-fat dressings, baked potatoes, chili, and chicken soft tacos are other good choices. If you must get a burger, choose the smallest size and be sure to omit the mayo. Get a baked potato or a salad with fat-free dressing on the side. Roast beef sandwiches with mustard or barbecue sauce are another option that is fairly low in fat. As for pizzas, choose plenty of vegetable toppings and skip the extra cheese. Even better, ask for *half* the cheese. If you want a meat topping, choose Canadian bacon or lean ham.

How high in fat can fast food get? A typical large cheeseburger with a mayonnaise-type dressing will contain 500 to 700 calories and 35 to 45 grams of fat. Double-meat burgers, of course, are even worse. Add a medium order of fries for about 350 calories and 18 grams of fat. Fried chicken and fish sandwiches tend to be a little lower than burgers, with 400 to 500 calories and 15 to 25 grams of fat. But some, like the Burger King Big Fish Sandwich and Chicken Sandwich, contain over 700 calories and 40 grams of fat. Are chicken nuggets any better? An average order will provide about 300 calories and 15 fat grams. As for breakfast choices, a sausage, egg, and cheese-stuffed breakfast biscuit or croissant will start your day with 500 calories and 35 to 40 grams of fat.

A final warning is in order regarding fast foods. Beware of seemingly innocent salads, like grilled chicken Caesar salads and taco salads. For instance, the Boston Market Chicken Caesar salad, which comes pretossed with an oily dressing and topped with fried croutons, contains 47 grams of fat and 670 calories. As for the taco salad, between the fried shell, meat, cheese, and sour cream, this creation can be loaded with fat and calories. In fact, the Taco Bell Taco Salad contains 840 calories and 52 grams of fat. It is best to avoid these two salads unless the menu specifically states they are low in fat. To help you avoid high-fat surprises, the following table lists some commonly available fast foods that are in the lower range of fat and calories.

Fast Foods Lowest in Calories and Fat

Fast Food	Calories	Fat	Sodium
BOSTON MARKET			
$1/4$ White Meat Chicken (no skin or wing)	160	3.5 g	350 mg
Skinless Rotisserie Turkey Breast	170	1 g	850 mg
Chicken Sandwich (no sauce or cheese)	430	4.5 g	910 mg
Turkey Sandwich (no sauce or cheese)	400	3.5 g	1,070 mg
Ham Sandwich (no sauce or cheese)	450	9 g	1,600 mg
Ham Turkey Club Sandwich (no sauce or cheese)	430	6 g	1,330 mg
Chicken Soup ($3/4$ cup)	80	3 g	470 mg
Whole Kernel Corn ($3/4$ cup)	180	4 g	170 mg
Fruit Salad ($3/4$ cup)	70	0.5 g	10 mg
New Potatoes ($3/4$ cup)	130	2.5 g	150 mg
Steamed Vegetables ($2/3$ cup)	35	0.5 g	35 mg
Zucchini Marinara ($3/4$ cup)	80	4 g	470 mg

Fast Food	Calories	Fat	Sodium
BURGER KING			
B.K. Broiler Chicken Sandwich (no mayo)	380	12 g	945 mg
Broiled Chicken Salad	190	8 g	500 mg
Garden Salad	100	5 g	110 mg
Side Salad	60	3 g	55 mg
Reduced-Calorie Light Italian Dressing	15	0.5 g	360 mg
CHICK-FIL-A [1]			
Chargrilled Chicken Sandwich	280	3 g	640 mg
Chargrilled Chicken Deluxe Sandwich	290	3 g	640 mg
Chicken Salad Sandwich on whole wheat	320	5 g	810 mg
Hearty Breast of Chicken Soup (cup)	110	1 g	760 mg
Chargrilled Chicken Garden Salad	170	3 g	650 mg
Chicken Salad Plate	290	5 g	570 mg
Tossed Salad	70	0 g	0 mg
Carrot Raisin Salad (small)	150	2 g	650 mg
Lite Italian Salad Dressing (3 tbsp)	20	1 g	770 mg
Lite Ranch (3 tbsp)	100	7 g	300 mg
Fat-Free Honey Mustard (3 tbsp)	70	0.5 g	230 mg
DOMINO'S PIZZA			
12-inch Hand-Tossed Cheese Pizza (2 slices)	347	10.7 g	723 mg
12-inch Hand-Tossed Ham Pizza (2 slices)	364	11.4 g	885 mg
12-inch Hand Tossed Veggie Pizza (2 slices)	356	11.4 g	723 mg
Fat-Free Ranch Dressing	40	0 g	560 mg
Large Garden Salad	39	0.5 g	26 mg
Light Italian Dressing	20	1 g	780 mg
HARDEE'S			
Pancakes (3) (plain)	280	2 g	890 mg
Grilled Chicken Sandwich	350	11 g	950 mg

[1] The nutrition information for Chick-Fil-A Chicken Salad Sandwich, Chicken Salad Plate, and Carrot Raisin Salad are based on the use of a *very small amount* of full-fat mayonnaise in the recipes. If the products seem to contain a good deal of mayonnaise at your particular restaurant, you should suspect that they contain more fat than what is listed.

Fast Food	Calories	Fat	Sodium
Regular Hamburger	270	11 g	670 mg
Hot Ham 'N' Cheese	310	12 g	1,410 mg
Mashed Potatoes (4 ounces)	70	<1 g	330 mg
Gravy (1.5 ounces)	20	<1 g	260 mg
Baked Beans (5 ounces)	170	1 g	600 mg
Grilled Chicken Salad	150	3 g	610 mg
Garden Salad	220	13 g	350 mg
Side Salad	25	<1 g	45 mg
Fat-Free French Dressing (2 ounces)	70	0 g	580 mg
Vanilla Cone	170	2 g	130 mg
Chocolate Cone	180	2 g	110 mg
Hot Fudge Sundae	290	6 g	310 mg
Strawberry Sundae	210	2 g	140 mg

KENTUCKY FRIED CHICKEN

	Calories	Fat	Sodium
Tender Roast Chicken breast (no skin)	169	4.3 g	797 mg
BBQ Chicken Sandwich	256	8 g	782 mg
BBQ Baked Beans (5.5 ounces)	190	3 g	760 mg
Corn on the Cob (5 ounces)	150	1.5 g	20 mg
Green Beans (4.7 ounces)	45	1.5 g	730 mg
Mean Greens (5.4 ounces)	70	3 g	650 mg
Mashed Potatoes With Gravy (4.8 ounces)	120	6 g	440 mg

MCDONALD'S

	Calories	Fat	Sodium
Small Hamburger (plain)	260	9 g	580 mg
Grilled Chicken Deluxe Sandwich (no mayo)	300	5 g	930 mg
Grilled Chicken Salad Deluxe	120	1.5 g	240 mg
Garden Salad	35	0 g	20 mg
Fat-Free Herb Vinaigrette Salad Dressing (1 packet)	50	0 g	330 mg
Egg McMuffin	290	12 g	710 mg
English Muffin	140	2 g	210 mg
Hotcakes (plain)	310	7 g	610 mg
Low-Fat Apple Bran Muffin	300	3 g	380 mg
1% Low-Fat Milk (8 ounces)	100	2.5 g	115 mg
Orange Juice (6 ounces)	80	0 g	20 mg
Vanilla Low-Fat Ice Cream Cone	150	4.5 g	75 mg

Fast Food	Calories	Fat	Sodium
SUBWAY [2]			
6-Inch Subs			
Veggie Delite™	237	3 g	593 mg
Turkey Breast	289	4 g	1,403 mg
Turkey Breast & Ham	295	5 g	1,361 mg
Ham	302	5 g	1,319 mg
Roast Beef	303	5 g	939 mg
Subway Club®	312	5 g	1,352 mg
Subway Seafood & Crab®	347	10 g	884 mg
Tuna	391	15 g	940 mg
B.L.T.	327	10 g	957 mg
Cold Cut Trio	378	13 g	1,412 mg
Roasted Chicken Breast	348	6 g	978 mg
Steak & Cheese*	398	10 g	1,117 mg
Subway Melt™*	382	12 g	1,746 mg
Deli Style Sandwiches			
Turkey Breast	235	4 g	944 mg
Ham	234	4 g	773 mg
Roast Beef	245	4 g	638 mg
Tuna	279	9 g	583 mg
Salads and Dressings			
Veggie Delite™	51	1 g	308 mg
Turkey Breast	102	2 g	1,117 mg
Subway Club®	126	3 g	1,067 mg
Roasted Chicken Breast	162	4 g	693 mg
Cold Cut Trio	191	11 g	1,127 mg
Roast Beef	117	3 g	654 mg
Ham	116	3 g	1,034 mg
Turkey Breast & Ham	109	3 g	1,076 mg
Steak & Cheese*	212	8 g	832 mg
B.L.T.	140	8 g	672 mg

[2] The nutrition information listed for Subway sandwiches and salads does not include dressing, oil, or mayonnaise. The nutritional information for sandwiches and salads includes cheese only on those items marked with an asterisk (*). (Two triangles of cheese will add 41 calories and 3 grams of fat.) The information listed for Seafood and Crab Salad and Tuna Salad products are based on the use of light mayonnaise in the recipe. Check with your individual restaurant to see if they use light mayonnaise in these menu items, as some restaurants use full-fat mayonnaise instead.

Fast Food	Calories	Fat	Sodium
Subway Melt™*	195	10 g	1,461 mg
Subway Seafood & Crab®	161	8 g	599 mg
Tuna	205	13 g	654 mg
Bread Bowl	330	4 g	760 mg
Fat-Free Italian dressing (1 tbsp)	5	0 g	152 mg
Fat-Free Ranch dressing (1 tbsp)	12	0 g	177 mg
Fat-Free French dressing (1 tbsp)	15	0 g	85 mg
TACO BELL			
Grilled Chicken Soft Taco	240	12 g	1,110 mg
Taco	180	10 g	330 mg
Soft Taco	220	10 g	580 mg
Grilled Steak Soft Taco	230	10 g	1,020 mg
Bean Burrito	380	12 g	1,110 mg
WENDY'S			
Grilled Chicken Sandwich	310	8 g	790 mg
Chili (small/8 ounces)	210	7 g	800 mg
Baked Potato (plain)	310	0 g	25 mg
Caesar Side Salad	110	4 g	620 mg
Side Salad	60	3 g	180 mg
Grilled Chicken Salad	200	8 g	720 mg
Grilled Chicken Caesar Salad	260	9 g	1,170 mg
Deluxe Garden Salad	110	6 g	350 mg
Fat-free French Dressing (2 tbsp)	35	0 g	150 mg
Reduced-Calorie Italian dressing (2 tbsp)	40	3 g	340 mg
Reduced-Fat Ranch Dressing (2 tbsp)	60	5 g	240 mg
Soft Breadstick	130	3 g	250 mg
Chicken Caesar Pita (no dressing)	420	11 g	1,150 mg
Classic Greek Pita (no dressing)	370	13 g	880 mg
Garden Ranch Chicken Pita (no dressing)	430	13 g	1,055 mg
Garden Veggie Pita (no dressing)	350	12 g	635 mg
WHATABURGER			
Pancakes (3)	259	5.8 g	842 mg
Syrup (1 packet)	180	0 g	50 mg
Egg Omelette Sandwich	288	12.8 g	602 mg
Grilled Chicken Sandwich (no mayo)	385	8.5 g	989 mg

Fast Food	Calories	Fat	Sodium
Chicken Fajita	272	6.7 g	691 mg
Beef Fajita	326	11.9 g	670 mg
Justaburger	276	11.3 g	578 mg
Baked Potato (plain)	310	0 g	23 mg
Grilled Chicken Salad	150	1.2 g	434 mg
Garden Salad	56	0.6 g	32 mg
Low-Fat Ranch Dressing (1 packet)	66	3.3 g	607 mg
Low-Fat Vinaigrette Dressing (1 packet)	37	1.8 g	896 mg

EATING IN THE AIR

Air travel can really sidetrack even the best of intentions to eat healthfully. Flights with long layovers or unexpected delays can leave you with so much time on your hands that you succumb to eating out of boredom. Flights at odd hours or with tight connections can mean a day of living on peanuts, sodas, and other junk food grabbed on the run. But don't despair. With just a little preparation, you can make it to your destination with your low-fat diet intact. Here are some ideas.

☐ Check your itinerary to see if a meal will be served on your flight. If so, call ahead to see if you can place a special meal request. Most airlines offer options such as low-fat meals, diabetic meals, cold seafood plates, fruit platters, and vegetarian meals. (Call at least twenty-four hours ahead to insure that your request is honored.)

☐ If no meals will be served on your flight, and you will not have any time to eat between flights, pack your own meal or snack and take it on board. Otherwise you will be starving by the time you reach your destination, and will be more likely to make poor food choices out of desperation.

☐ If you want a snack while on board, request pretzels instead of peanuts, and choose mineral water with lime, tomato juice, or fruit juice for a beverage.

☐ Between the dry cabin air and reduced access to water, it's easy to become dehydrated during air travel. Keep your own bottle of water handy, and drink often. This will also help prevent you from snacking when you are really just thirsty.

☐ If you have a layover in an airport, there are plenty of low-fat choices for meals and snacks these days. For a quick snack, you can almost always find delis and coffee shops that sell cartons of low-fat yogurt, fresh fruit cups, bagels, and soups. Low-fat frozen yogurt and soft pretzel stands are also conveniently located in most airports. Salads with low-fat dressing and lean meat sandwiches on whole grain bread are easily found in most airports when you want a light and healthy meal. When you have more time, most major airports have full-service restaurants, including some national chains that offer lighter fare.

☐ Keep snacks such as low-fat granola bars, small boxes of raisins, and fresh fruit on hand in case you have an unexpected delay at odd hours.

☐ Take some reading material or work with you to fill long flights, layovers, and unexpected delays. This is also a good time to catch up on letter writing or handicrafts such as needlepoint. Keeping busy is the best way to prevent eating out of boredom.

EATING ON THE ROAD

Whether you are traveling for work or pleasure, car trips offer more freedom than other forms of travel, giving you the opportunity to shop for restaurants, to pack a cooler, or to stop at a grocery store for healthy snacks. Here are some ideas for making the most of meals on the road.

☐ Choose meals from fast food restaurants, sandwich shops, and full-service restaurants using the guidelines presented on pages 150 to 164.

☐ Instead of opting for restaurant fare, consider stopping at a grocery store. Grocery stores often have delis where you can have a sandwich made to order with lean meat, vegetables, and whole grain bread. Many also have complete salad bars where you can compile a low-fat salad. While you're there, stock up on bottled water, fresh fruit, baby carrots, low-fat granola bars, and other healthful snacks.

☐ Keep a cooler in your car and stock it with yogurt, sandwich fixings, and beverages. Then, weather permitting, find a rest stop and enjoy a picnic lunch instead of going to a restaurant. This will give you a nice break and a chance to walk and stretch, as well.

☐ Keep plenty of water handy so that you don't find yourself snacking when you are really just thirsty.

☐ For breakfast, keep in mind that cereal, bagels, and other foods can be purchased at a local grocery store while on the road, and later eaten in your hotel room.

☐ If you have the continental breakfast at a hotel, choose fresh fruit; low-fat milk; and whole wheat or rye toast, bagels, or English muffins with jam instead of butter. Skip the donuts, pastries, and high-fat muffins.

EATING AT THE OFFICE

Most people spend close to a third of their life at work, and from midmorning donut breaks, to goodies brought in by coworkers, to desktop candy jars, to lunches out, the workplace abounds with occupational eating hazards. Here are some simple strategies to help you avoid fat traps at the office.

☐ Watch the coffee. A couple of cups of coffee a day is not problem for most people. And without the creamer, coffee is calorie-free. Add cream, though, and the calories can add up. Just one tablespoon of cream contains 30 calories and 2.9 grams of fat.

Half-and-half is only a little better, with 20 calories and 1.7 grams of fat per table-spoon. Fat-free nondairy creamers will provide 10 to 20 calories per tablespoon. The flavored sweetened versions, such as amaretto or Irish cream, can contain even more. People who drink several cups of coffee per day, each containing 2 tablespoons of creamer, can get an extra 100 to 200 calories per day that they don't even think about. Add a few teaspoons of sugar to each cup, and you could pick up another 100 calories. This may not seem like much until you realize that consuming an extra 100 calories per day will cause you to gain 10 pounds in a year! Your most healthful choice for lightening coffee is instant nonfat dry milk powder or evaporated skimmed milk. Both are fat-free and low in calories, and will add some calcium to your diet.

☐ Skip the midmorning donuts. Most people need a break by midmorning, and many fill that break with food—even when they're not hungry. Don't forget that just one glazed donut will add about 250 calories to your day. Iced donuts and Danish pastries are even worse. If you need a midmorning snack, bring your own, choosing something healthful like fresh fruit, baby carrots, low-fat string cheese, or nonfat yogurt. If possible, use your break to take a short walk. Walking is far more rejuvenating than a sugary snack.

☐ Eat a balanced lunch. Many people on low-fat diets fall into the habit of eating a simple high-carbohydrate lunch, like a baked potato, pasta with marinara sauce, or even a bag of popcorn. While low in fat, these meals are unbalanced, and will leave you feeling tired and sleepy by midafternoon. The reason? When eaten alone—that is, without any protein foods—high-carbohydrate foods raise brain levels of serotonin, a neurotransmitter that makes you feel relaxed and sleepy. To make matters worse, when midafternoon fatigue sets in, many people begin snacking in an effort to boost energy levels. Of course, high-fat lunches like a cheeseburger and fries will also make you feel tired, since fatty foods sit in your stomach for a long time and require much of your energy to be diverted to digestion.

If you want to remain alert and energetic throughout the afternoon, have a balanced low-fat meal at lunch, including a low-fat protein source, a grain or starch, and plenty of vegetables and/or fruits. A salad topped with fat-free cheese and chickpeas, some grilled fish with a plain baked potato and a salad or vegetables, or a lean meat or tuna sandwich and a piece of fruit will do the trick. If you need to remain extra alert in the afternoon, try an energizing "power" lunch. In other words, eat just the lean protein and vegetables, and save the starch for dinner. (If you have diabetes, always check with your physician or nutritionist before altering the carbohydrate content of your meals.)

☐ Steer clear of desktop candy jars. A piece here and a piece there can really add up by the end of the day. Everyone knows that chocolates and bite-size candy bars are high in fat and calories, but what about fat-free candies like jelly beans? At 800 calories per cup, jelly beans are pure sugar and no bargain.

☐ Don't feel pressured to purchase candy, cookies, or other goodies from coworkers who are selling these products for fundraisers. If you buy it, you'll probably end up eating it.

☐ Keep a water bottle on your desk. People often snack when they are really just thirsty. Staying properly hydrated is your best defense.

☐ Keep office parties in perspective. Unfortunately, many people work in an office where people find every excuse to bring in birthday cakes and other goodies, and to arrange potluck breakfasts or lunches. When these situations are unavoidable, let the strategies for handling parties on pages 173 and 174 guide you in making the best possible choices. Better yet, suggest alternatives, like sending out for frozen yogurt or giving movie tickets for birthdays and other celebrations. When having potluck meals at the office, bring something healthy so that you know there will be at least one thing you can eat without blowing your fat budget.

MUNCHING AT THE MOVIES

Movies and popcorn just seem to go together. Thank goodness popcorn is a healthy snack, right? It depends on how it's made. And at movie theaters, the overwhelming majority of popcorn is popped in some kind of fat—either coconut oil, vegetable oil, or solid shortening.

This adds about 20 to 25 grams of fat to a small (6- to 8-cup) serving of naturally fat-free popcorn. Add the buttery topping, and the fat grams will almost double. In the interest of health, some theaters have switched from coconut oil and hydrogenated shortenings to liquid canola oil for popping their corn. This a healthier option, since canola oil won't clog your arteries. However, the total calories and fat grams in the popcorn will be exactly the same—about 330 to 440 calories and 20 to 25 grams of fat per small serving.

How can you have your popcorn and eat it too? Some theaters do offer air-popped corn as an alternative to the traditional high-fat version. And some theaters are starting to sell other lighter snacks, such as hot pretzels and low-fat frozen yogurt bars. If your theater doesn't offer any low-fat snack options, consider bringing your own munchies. A snack-sized bag of low-fat microwave popcorn is perfect for one person. Or pop a standard-sized bag and share with a friend. As long as you are not obvious about carting in your own snacks (discreetly hide them under your jacket or in a large purse), most theaters will have no problem with this.

SNACKING AT SPORTS EVENTS

Here's one area where the pickings are still pretty slim for fat-conscious folks. Whether your spectator sport is baseball, football, hockey, or basketball, your snack choices are pretty limited. Full-fat hot dogs, fried tortilla chips covered with cheese, greasy pizza, oil-popped popcorn, and high-fat peanuts still reign as the primary snack offerings at sporting events. Fortunately, a few low-fat snacks such as soft pretzels with mustard and frozen yogurt are typically offered, as well. Additionally, food vendors vary from stadium to stadium and city to city. In progressive communities, you may even find vendors selling items like shish kabobs, grilled chicken sandwiches, and veggie burgers. The following table lists the fat and calorie contents of some common stadium snacks.

Calories and Fat in Selected Stadium Snacks

Snack Food	Calories	Fat
Hot dog, plain (2-ounce frank with bun)	294	18.3 g
Nachos (2 ounces chips with 2 ounces cheese)	466	28 g
Peanuts (¹/4 cup shelled)	213	18 g
Pizza, pepperoni (1 medium slice)	230	11 g
Popcorn (6 cups, unbuttered)	330	19 g
Popcorn (6 cups, buttered)	430	30 g
Pretzel, soft (2 ounce)	196	1.7 g
Yogurt, low-fat frozen (1 cup)	207	1.6 g

ENJOYING PARTIES AND HOLIDAYS

For most of us, party food spells fun and festivity—and fat. Cheesy dips, fried chips, greasy meatballs, and other high-fat fare make most special occasions a nightmare for anyone who's trying to eat healthfully.

If special occasions were few and far between, a once-in-a-while fat overdose would not be a problem. But when you add up all the birthdays, anniversaries, weddings, and other gatherings that crop up during the year, you may find that the amount of fat you get from parties is not a trivial matter. Besides, once you discover how delicious low-fat eating can be, and how great you look and feel on a slimmed-down diet, you will want to eat this way all year round. The remainder of the chapter will guide you through a variety of festivities, from parties that you give yourself, to parties that you attend, to the winter round of holiday festivities.

Hosting a Party

When you are the host or hostess, there is plenty you can do to get the fat out of party favorites. Nonfat and low-fat cheeses, nonfat sour cream and mayonnaise, ultra-lean lunchmeats, baked chips, and a multitude of other products can help take the fat out of your celebrations and get-togethers. Chapter 5 offers a wealth of ideas for using these low-fat products in your favorite recipes, and Chapter 6 presents recipes for a variety of fat-free party-perfect treats. You'll be amazed at the big fat difference a few simple ingredient substitutions can make in traditional party favorites. For instance, a bowl of dip made with a cup of full-fat mayonnaise gets 1,582 calories and 186 fat grams from the mayonnaise alone. Prepare the same dip with a light mayonnaise, and you will cut the fat and calories by 50 to 80 percent. Use a nonfat mayonnaise, and you will eliminate all of the fat and 90 percent of the calories!

Attending a Party

What if someone else is doing the cooking? Your best defense is to know which party foods are lowest in calories and fat, and to choose these most often. Steamed seafood platters with cocktail sauce are an excellent choice. From the cold cut platter, choose sliced turkey, ham, and roast beef. And, of course, the fresh fruit and vegetable platter is a great choice—provided you avoid the fatty dip that may accompany it. Choose pretzels, crackers, and breads over fried potato chips and fried tortilla chips. And, by all means, avoid the nut dish. Just a quarter cup of nuts has close to 200 calories and 18 grams of fat. Use the following guidelines to help you enjoy parties without blowing your fat or calorie budgets.

□ *Plan ahead.* If you know that you will be going to a party, work it into your daily meal plan. Save a third to a fourth of that day's calorie allotment for a cocktail party, and a third to a half of your allotment for a dinner party. Avoid going out for dinner after a cocktail party, as you will almost certainly overshoot your food limit for the day. Heavy hors d'oeuvres should be considered dinner. (To learn about turning a cocktail party into dinner, see the inset on page 175.)

□ *Don't starve yourself.* If you go to your party feeling ravenous, you will most likely overeat. Don't starve yourself all day in anticipation of the goodies ahead. Instead, eat a light breakfast and lunch, and save some calories for the evening.

□ *Eat only special foods.* Don't waste fat and calories on ordinary snack and party foods, like chips and dips. Concentrate on foods that aren't usually available, and then eat them only in moderation.

□ *Eat slowly.* By eating slowly, you will feel more satisfied with less food. (After twenty minutes of eating, the body signals a feeling of fullness to the brain.)

□ *Remember the law of diminishing returns.* The more you eat of something, the less pleasure you receive. For example, that first bite of cheesecake is the best, because the taste is so new. As you continue to eat, the pleasure diminishes. So eat just a bite or two, and receive 90 percent of the pleasure for only 10 percent of the fat and calories!

□ *Don't set yourself up for failure.* Make a conscious effort to position yourself away from the hors d'oeuvres. This will prevent you from munching away as you chat with others.

□ *Beware of the bubbly.* Alcohol contains almost as many calories as fat does. Combine it with creamy or sweet mixers, and you get even more calories. For instance, a small (6-ounce) white Russian contains about 315 calories and 14 grams of fat. Another problem is that alcohol lowers your inhibitions, possibly making you careless about food choices. What can you do? Sip a wine spritzer, or mix the liquor with water, soda, or a diet beverage. Then alternate alcoholic drinks with glasses of water. Or simply drink club soda or another nonalcoholic beverage instead of the alcohol, and spend more of your calorie budget on party foods.

□ *Offer to bring something to the party.* This way you will know that there will be at least one item you can enjoy without blowing your fat budget. Chapter 6 offers a selection of low-fat party-pleasing appetizers that are so delicious, no one will even guess that they're healthful.

How to Turn a Cocktail Party Into Dinner

If the host of your next party has not yet discovered the joys of low-fat cuisine, you will probably be faced with a tempting table of high-fat hors d'oeuvres. Heavy hors d'oeuvres can and should be considered dinner for anyone who is watching his or her waistline. Even then, these appetizing tidbits must be selected properly to provide a balanced meal that doesn't quickly outstrip a reasonable allotment of calories and fat. Here are some guidelines:

☐ Begin with an "entrée"—some high-protein appetizers such as steamed shrimp, or some slices of turkey breast, roast beef, or ham. Steer clear of the cheese cubes, which will provide close to 10 grams of fat per ounce (a couple of bites). Eat in moderation. There's more to come!

☐ A well-balanced meal must include some vegetables, so move over to the vegetable tray for your next course. Try to use a minimal amount of dip.

☐ For your bread choice, have some whole grain crackers or breads if available. Or have some pretzels, which are usually standard fare on an hors d'oeuvres table.

☐ Fruit lends refreshing balance to the meal, and adds no fat, so have a generous serving of melon, pineapple, berries, or other fresh fruits.

☐ For your beverage, pour yourself a glass of club soda or spring water, or choose a diet soft drink.

☐ For dessert, serve yourself a small portion of something decadent that you really want. Then enjoy it!

So the next time you're invited to a party, don't despair. You don't have to blow your fat budget in order to enjoy yourself. Just pretend that you've been invited out to dinner, and serve yourself a meal that's high on satisfaction and low on guilt.

Handling the Holidays

Holidays can be difficult times for fat-fighters, since each holiday is centered on its own traditional foods—most of which are loaded with fat and calories. Overindulging is even *expected* on the holidays, and most people are willing to make an exception for the day and go "all out" with food and drink.

November and December are especially difficult months for those of us who are watching calories and fat grams. 'Tis the season for family feasts, office parties, and open houses. For two months, we are faced with every culinary temptation imaginable, and the whole country seems to develop an eat-now-pay-later mentality. It's not unusual for people to gain seven to twelve pounds during the winter holidays. And despite good intentions come January 2, many people never are able to lose the full amount they gained.

Fortunately, the situation is far from hopeless. It is possible to enjoy all the festivities—including the special foods that help make the season enjoyable—and still stay within the boundaries of a reasonable diet. So take heart, and use the following strategies to help maintain some semblance of sanity during the festive season.

☐ *Prepare yourself for the party circuit.* During the winter holidays, you may be invited to a party almost every day. Use the strategies presented on pages 173 and 174 to help you plan ahead for parties and to make wise, but still enjoyable, food choices.

☐ *Spend your calorie and fat budgets wisely.* During the holidays, food is everywhere—the office, parties, open houses, formal dinners, and church and school functions. This is definitely the time to be discriminating. Don't waste fat and calories on ordinary junk foods that are available all year round. Instead, concentrate on foods that aren't usually available. Then choose your very favorites, and enjoy them in moderation.

☐ *Watch out for food gifts.* The holidays bring out the baker and candy maker in many people. And, of course, they just love to prepare their most calorie-, sugar-, and fat-laden treats to give out as gifts. Have just a little, if you like, working the foods into your daily calorie and fat allotment. Then, as the food gifts pile up, consider giving them to a homeless shelter. And don't feel bad about throwing away excess goodies—it's better that they wind up in the garbage than around your waistline. If you like to give gifts of food, try putting together a fresh fruit basket or a selection of gourmet teas and coffees. If you're feeling more creative, make up some canisters of hot cocoa mix, jars of homemade jam, or attractive bottles of flavored vinegars. Gifts like these, which do not require immediate consumption, are always welcome.

☐ *Modify your favorite holiday recipes.* Just about any holiday recipe can be made with less fat, sugar, and calories, and remain every bit as enjoyable. See Chapter 5 and the following section, "Trimming the Fat from Your Holiday Feasts," for ideas.

☐ *Enlist the help of others.* No one wants to put on excess pounds during the holidays, so enlist the help of friends, family, and coworkers. You'll then be able to help one another plan more healthful menus and eat within reason.

Trimming the Fat From Your Holiday Feasts

If you look at holiday dinners past, it's easy to see why we all feel the need to start a diet the morning after. Take Thanksgiving, for instance. The parade of tempting dishes often begins even before dinner with several appetizers, perhaps accompanied by wine. Then comes the turkey, and possibly a ham. With the turkey is served three or four different starches—stuffing, mashed potatoes, sweet potatoes, and rolls, for instance—as well as two or more vegetables. And, of course, there's cranberry sauce.

Naturally, the turkey, stuffing, and potatoes are topped with fat-laden gravy. And last, but not least, comes a fabulous selection of rich desserts. Even if you insist on fairly small portions, you're likely to use up an entire day's calorie allotment on a dinner like this. You're also likely to feel uncomfortably full at meal's end.

However, it really is possible to enjoy Thanksgiving and other holidays and still eat healthfully. Realize that holiday meals can be a lot simpler than they usually are, but every bit as enjoyable and well-balanced. For instance, roast turkey with stuffing and gravy with one other starch—either sweet potatoes or mashed potatoes, for instance—a salad, a vegetable, and dessert, make a well-balanced and satisfying meal. What can you do about those fat-laden holiday recipes? Keep them, but give them slimming makeovers. Here are some ideas for trimming the fat from holiday feasts.

Entrées

Turkey is an ideal low-fat first course for Thanksgiving, Christmas, and Easter. To keep it this way, buy a fresh, unbasted turkey instead of the prebasted kind, which has been injected with a mixture of oil and salty broth. Baste your bird with broth or wine instead of fat, and cover it with foil during cooking to seal in moisture. (Remove the foil during the last thirty minutes to promote browning.) To make delicious fat-free gravy, first defat the pan drippings using the tips on page 88. You can also make moist and delicious stuffing without the usual butter or margarine by following the guideline on page 75.

For a change of pace, serve lean ham or roasted pork tenderloins filled with a savory stuffing for your holiday dinner. For warm weather holidays like the Fourth of July, Memorial Day, and Labor Day, break out the grill and cook up some 95-percent lean ground beef burgers, shish kabobs, skinless chicken, fish, London broil, or pork tenderloin. Use marinades and rubs (pages 89 and 92) to add delicious flavor to grilled lean meats, chicken, and fish.

Side dishes

Moisten your mashed potatoes with evaporated skimmed milk, nonfat margarine, plain nonfat yogurt, or nonfat sour cream. When making casseroles, use nonfat or low-fat cheeses, low-fat cream soups, and nonfat sour cream. Lighten your salads with low- and no-fat mayonnaise, nonfat sour cream, and fat-free salad dressings.

Desserts

Use evaporated skimmed milk in pumpkin pies; substitute egg whites for whole eggs; and reduce the sugar by 25 percent. Choose fruit-based desserts, like cobblers and fruit crisps, over gooey cakes and pastries.

Although eating away from home presents a special challenge to fat-fighters, as you've seen, it is possible to follow a healthy diet in virtually any situation. The secret is to anticipate the special event—whether a lavish holiday party or a simple lunch with friends—and to have ready the strategies that will allow you to achieve your goals. Then sit back and enjoy the many benefits and pleasures of fat-free living.

8. Exercise – The Other Secret of Living Fat-Free

E veryone knows that exercise is good for you, but over the past few years, research has proven exercise to be even more important for promoting optimal health than anyone had ever realized. Unfortunately, more than 60 percent of adults do not exercise regularly, and 25 percent do not exercise at all. This is a shame, because even moderate amounts of exercise can provide tremendous benefits.

Exercise enhances a fat-free lifestyle in many ways. First, if you are trying to lose weight, exercise will support your low-fat diet by directly burning calories. Exercise will also help you lose fat and build muscle. And since muscle needs more calories to maintain itself than fat does, over time, exercise will increase your metabolic rate. Stressed out? Exercise is one of the very best ways to cope with stress—and this, too, can help you control your weight. As you may know, when stressed, people often revert to eating fatty foods and to snacking excessively. If you have a regular exercise program, you will deal with stress better and be much less likely to use food as a coping mechanism. (See the inset on page 180 for more on stress and exercise.) Finally, exercise will help you make the most of your low-fat diet by providing added protection against health problems like heart disease and diabetes. For all these reasons and many more, exercise is an essential part of living fat-free.

Must you spend grueling hours in the gym or on a treadmill to get the benefits of exercise? No. Even moderate amounts of exercise can provide great benefits. And exercise doesn't have to be a chore to be effective. The rest of this chapter will provide plenty of ideas for making exercise an enjoyable part of your fat-free lifestyle. As you will see, done properly and consistently, exercise can be a highly effective "secret weapon" in your fight against fat.

HOW MUCH IS ENOUGH?

When some people begin an exercise program, they work out so strenuously that they quickly exhaust themselves and abandon their regimen. Others exercise so little that the benefits are negligible. Just how much exercise is necessary for good health? There are actually two different sets of recommendations for exercise. The first and most basic recommendation, issued by the Surgeon General of the United States in

Exercise—The Best Medicine for Stress

Since the beginning of time, stress has been a part of everyday life. However, for many thousands of years, the stress that people faced was mostly physical. Protecting oneself from wild animals, wars, and other threats to daily survival were the norm. Today's stressors, on the other hand, are mostly psychological in nature—competing in the professional world and dealing with financial pressures, for instance. Let's take a look at how the body reacts when a person faces stress, and how these reactions apply to today's world.

When a person first perceives a threat or stressor, the body responds by secreting hormones and by activating nerves that prepare the body to fight or run away. This is called the fight-or-flight response. Your muscles tense so that you can have maximum strength ready, your heart rate and breathing speed up to supply extra oxygen to muscles, and blood sugar and fat levels rise to provide fuels to exercising muscles.

As you can see, when faced with a physical threat, the fight-or-flight response serves you well. However, when faced with a psychological stressor, the body's reaction to stress can actually be a handicap. Why? Like physical stressors, psychological stressors prepare the body for physical motion—fight or flight. But when you experience a psychological stressor and you don't do anything physical to compensate, your muscles remain tense, your heart rate and breathing remain elevated, and you have elevated blood levels of sugar and fat. This situation leaves you feeling anxious and puts you at risk for heart disease and other health problems.

Unfortunately, many people reach for food—especially fatty, sugary foods—when they feel stressed. While this may bring about short-term relief, it only makes the problem worse in the long run by contributing to obesity and poor health.

What's a healthier way to deal with stress? Exercise. Since stress prepares the body for physical motion, exercise allows the stress to be released. As you work out, you will actually feel the stress leaving your body. Your tense muscles will relax again, the accumulated sugar and fat in your blood will burn, and your heart rate and breathing will return to normal. This is why people who have a regular exercise program— whether it's walking, biking, weight lifting, dancing, or playing a sport— cope better with stress. Regular exercise will also make you much less likely to fall prey to stress-induced eating, helping you stay on course with your healthy diet.

July 1996, is aimed at reducing the risk for disease and increasing longevity. If you are not used to exercising, this is the place to start. What does this basic exercise prescription entail? At the very minimum, you should exercise enough to burn 150 calories per day, or about 1,000 calories per week. This modest amount of exercise will cut your risk of heart disease by 50 percent, and your risk of high blood pressure, diabetes, and colon cancer by 30 percent.

How much exercise must you do to burn 150 calories? About thirty minutes of an activity such as brisk walking, dancing, or biking will do the trick for most people. Activities like gardening, yard work, washing the car, and heavy housework can also figure into your exercise allotment. It's really pretty easy to expend 150 calories per day with exercise, but when you consider that many people hire others to do their housework and yard work, take the car to a drive-through car wash, sit behind a desk all day at work, and have no formal exercise program, you can see why 60 percent of all adults do not engage in even this minimum amount of activity. The following table lists some activities that will burn 150 calories.

30 Ways to Burn 150 Calories

Activity	Time Required to Expend 150 Calories
Sports Activities	
Aerobic dancing (moderate intensity)	21 minutes
Aerobic dancing (high intensity)	16 minutes
Ballroom dancing	43 minutes
Basketball	16 minutes
Biking (10 miles per hour)	22 minutes
Canoeing (leisure)	50 minutes
Canoeing (racing)	21 minutes
Golf (pulling clubs)	26 minutes
Jumping rope (70 per minute)	14 minutes
Racquetball	13 minutes
Running (9-minute miles)	11 minutes
Running (6-minute miles)	9 minutes
Scuba diving	11 minutes
Swimming (breast stroke)	14 minutes
Tennis (singles)	20 minutes
Volleyball	44 minutes
Walking	27 minutes
Weight lifting (circuit training)	26 minutes
Housework	
Mopping floors	36 minutes
Scrubbing floors	20 minutes
Vacuuming floors	48 minutes
Window cleaning	38 minutes

Yard Work	
Chopping and stacking fire wood	25 minutes
Digging trenches	15 minutes
Hoeing	24 minutes
House painting	29 minutes
Mowing (push mower)	20 minutes
Raking	40 minutes
Washing and waxing car	45 minutes
Weeding	30 minutes

*Calories expended are based on a body weight of 150 pounds. People who weigh more will burn proportionately more calories than the table lists, and people who weigh less will burn proportionately fewer calories.

If you make exercise part of your family and social life, you can easily meet the goal of exercising away 150 calories a day. For instance, instead of sharing time with a friend by meeting for dinner, take an hour-long walk or bike ride together. Take your dog for a long walk at the end of the day to unwind and reduce stress, or get out and play a game of basketball with the kids. Plan a family hike or a biking or canoe trip on the weekend instead of going to a movie. Plant a vegetable or flower garden.

You can also increase the time you spend exercising by increasing your routine exercise—that is, the incidental exercise you do over the course of the day. For instance, try parking a little farther from your destination so that you will have to walk a greater distance. If you live only a couple of miles from work, consider walking or biking instead of driving. And take the stairs at work rather than the elevator. Little things like these can really add up over a period of time. Besides improvements in blood sugar, blood pressure, and overall health, the calories burned in exercise can add up to significant weight loss. Exercising away an extra 150 calories per day will cause you to lose 15 pounds by the end of the year!

Of course, the guideline for burning 150 calories per day with exercise is the *minimum* needed to achieve health benefits. Twice this amount would be an even better goal and would provide even greater benefits. This brings us to the second recommendation for exercise. For maximum fat-burning and health benefits, the American College of Sports Medicine recommends that you expand on the Surgeon General's guideline to develop a well-rounded program that includes both aerobic and strength-training exercises. The next sections look at the basics of these forms of exercise and describe the additional health benefits they provide.

THE BENEFITS OF AEROBIC EXERCISE

Aerobic exercise encompasses a wide variety of low- to moderate-intensity activities, including walking, running, biking, racquet sports, swimming, and dancing. These forms of exercise are fueled mostly by fat, which can be burned only when there is an adequate supply of oxygen present in the exercising muscles. Thus, during aerobic exercise, your heart and lungs deliver oxygen to exercising muscles. When you engage in this type of exercise consistently, your cardiovascular system becomes stronger and more efficient at delivering oxygen. This, in turn, greatly reduces your risk for a number of health problems. Some specific benefits that occur with aerobic exercise include:

☐ Your heart becomes larger and stronger, and can pump more blood with each beat. As a result, your pulse rate slows. (Pulse rate changes provide a convenient way to measure your training improvements.)

☐ Your blood volume increases, enabling your blood to carry more oxygen.

☐ Your blood pressure falls as blood flows more easily through your veins and arteries.

☐ Your blood levels of cholesterol and triglycerides drop, your HDL cholesterol levels rise, and your risk for heart disease greatly declines.

☐ Your lungs gain strength and endurance so that breathing becomes more efficient.

☐ The muscles throughout your body become firmer and stronger.

☐ Your muscles develop more fat-burning enzymes, and become more efficient at burning fat both during exercise and at rest.

☐ Your muscles become more sensitive to insulin, which helps keep blood sugar levels under control and reduces the risk for diabetes.

☐ Your immune system becomes stronger, reducing your risk for all kinds of illness.

To obtain the maximum health benefits of aerobic exercise, you need to engage in a minimum of twenty minutes of sustained aerobic activity at least three times a week, and you need to exercise at the appropriate intensity, which can be determined on the basis of your target heart rate. The target heart rate is the heart rate at which exercise is strenuous enough to push the heart, but not strain it. Exercising at this rate will allow you to gradually improve your aerobic fitness level.

To determine your target heart rate, first subtract your age from 220. This provides an estimate of the maximum heart rate for a person your age. Next, multiply your maximum heart rate by 65 percent to get the lower end of your target heart rate. For instance, if you are forty years old, your target heart rate will be 117 (220 - 40 = 180, and 180 x 0.65 = 117).

When you first begin your fitness program, a slow pace will push your heart to the target rate. As your fitness level improves, you will have to work at a faster pace to reach your target heart rate. If after a while you wish to increase your exercise intensity, you can work up to a target heart rate that equals 85 percent of your maximum heart rate. For a forty-year-old, this would be a pulse rate of 153 (220 - 40 =

Exercise Intensity and Fat Burning

Will you burn more fat walking for thirty minutes or running for thirty minutes? This is a common topic of conversation among exercisers, for it is widely believed that low-intensity exercises like walking burn more body fat than higher-intensity exercises like running. This is only partly true, and can be a misleading assumption. Here's why.

During all kinds of exercise, working muscles burn a mixture of fat and carbohydrate. For a low-intensity exercise like walking, the fuel mixture is about 70 percent fat and about 30 percent carbohydrate. For a high-intensity exercise like running, the proportions are just about reversed. Why? While walking, a person is able to breathe deeply and therefore deliver plenty of oxygen to exercising muscles. On the other hand, when running, breathing becomes labored, and less oxygen is able to reach exercising muscles. Since muscles need oxygen to burn fat, a walker burns a higher proportion of fat during exercise than a runner.

However, this is only part of the story. If you are trying to lose body fat, the total number of calories burned during exercise is more important than the intensity of the exercise. Here's why. If a 150-pound person walks for thirty minutes, he will burn about 162 calories. If he is using a fuel mixture of 70 percent fat and 30 percent carbohydrate, this amounts to 113 fat calories and 49 carbohydrate calories. If that same person runs for thirty minutes, he will burn about 393 calories. If he is using a fuel mixture of 30 percent fat and 70 percent carbohydrate, this amounts to 118 fat calories and 275 carbohydrate calories. As you can see, about the same amount of fat is being burned during each activity. But the more important factor is that the runner is burning more total calories. And as with diet, calories are the most important factor that determines your body fat stores. As long as the runner does not increase his caloric intake, he will have to burn some of his body fat *later* that day to make up for the extra calories lost during the run.

The bottom line is that you shouldn't get too caught up trying to figure out how much fat you will burn during exercise. Just pick an exercise that you like, and perform it long enough to burn a significant number of calories. If you burn more calories than you eat, you will lose body fat. It's that simple!

180, and 180 x .85 = 153). Be aware that certain blood pressure and heart medications can affect your heart rate, so if you take these or any other medications, you must check with your physician before starting an exercise program.

THE BENEFITS OF STRENGTH TRAINING

"Use it or lose it" aptly describes what happens to muscle mass as people age. And it's not just the elderly who suffer from muscle loss. For most people, the process starts in their twenties. To make matters worse, as people lose muscle over the years, they usually gain fat. What impact does this change in body composition have on your health? You lose strength, your bones get smaller and weaker, blood sugar levels rise, and blood cholesterol and triglycerides rise while HDL cholesterol levels decline. On top of all this, your metabolic rate drops so that you burn fewer calories and gain body fat more easily, which helps perpetuate the process. All of these occurrences have long been attributed to "normal" aging—a notion that infuriates exercise physiologists, who know that a large portion of these changes can actually be attributed to simple inactivity.

The good news is that you don't have to become a victim of the "normal" aging process. By strength training for just forty-five minutes two or three times a week, you can retard and even reverse much of the physical decline that most people experience as they age.

What is strength training? It is any exercise that makes muscles work against some kind of resistance—for instance, lifting weights or calisthenics like push-ups and pull-ups. If you have been sedentary for a while, a good way to start building muscles is with a body-toning class that uses free weights, exercise rubber bands, or resistance tubes. Activities like chopping wood and pushing a lawn mower can also help build muscles.

Must you join a gym to participate in a strength-training program? No. But many people opt to work out at a good gym because of the equipment and supervision that it can provide. A word of caution is in order, though. Don't rush into spending a lot of money on a gym membership until you are sure that this is what you want. Instead, see if you can purchase a short-term membership at a club, as this will allow you to evaluate the equipment and personnel before making a costly commitment. Likewise, don't spend a lot of money on home exercise equipment until you are sure you will use it.

One inexpensive option for people who are just beginning to strength train is a body-toning class that lets you pay as you go. Once you have mastered this level of strength training, you can progress to more challenging activities, like weight training. Yet another option is to do some calisthenics or exercises with free weights at home. When used in combination with regular activities like mowing the lawn, heavy yard work, and gardening, this can be enough to keep your muscles strong. Whatever you decide to do, as you progress in your strength-training program, the following benefits may be expected.

☐ Your bones become stronger and denser and less likely to fracture, and your risk of osteoporosis greatly declines.

☐ As you build muscle mass, your metabolic rate increases, causing you to burn more calories. This, in turn, makes it easier to lose body fat.

☐ Your body becomes firmer and denser. As you gain muscle and lose fat, you may notice that your clothes fit more loosely without there being a change in your body weight. This occurs because muscle weighs more than fat. If your primary goal is weight loss, don't get discouraged if you do not lose weight as quickly as you expected. Let your appearance be your guide, and further monitor your results by tracking changes in your body measurements or the percentage of body fat.

☐ Your tendons and joints become stronger and more elastic, enabling you to perform all activities more easily and with less risk of injury.

☐ Your muscles become more sensitive to insulin, helping you keep blood sugar levels under control and reduce the risk for diabetes.

Exercise Tips for Travelers

Traveling presents a real challenge for anyone who's trying to maintain a healthy diet and exercise regimen. As a result, many people tend to gain weight when they travel. Even worse, the disruption of their routine often makes it hard for them to get back on track when they return home. But as you learned in Chapter 7, travel does not have to disrupt your diet, and the same is true of travel and exercise. In fact, traveling can offer many new exercise adventures that will both enliven your vacation and tide you over until you return home and get back to your normal routine. Here are some ideas:

☐ If your hotel is located in a safe area, go for a walk or jog. This is a great way to see the city.

☐ Ask the hotel staff to recommend a restaurant that is a fifteen- to thirty-minute walk away. Again, this is a great way to see the local sights.

☐ Walk as much as possible on your sightseeing ventures. In addition, try to plan hikes, bicycle rides, canoe trips, tennis games, and other activities as part of your travel plans.

☐ Most hotels have swimming pools, and many hotels offer exercise rooms with weights, treadmills, and/or stationery bikes. Take advantage of these facilities.

☐ When possible, use the stairs in your hotel rather than the elevator.

☐ Before leaving on your vacation, use a cassette tape to record your favorite exercise class. Then work out to the tape when you're away.

☐ Become familiar with exercise rubber bands or resistance tubes, as these can be used anywhere.

☐ Check local gyms to see if they have walk-in rates or will honor your own gym membership at their facility.

☐ Wear your walking shoes when traveling by air. Then, if you have time, walk between terminals to catch flights instead of taking the moving sidewalk. If you have a long layover, use the time to walk around the airport.

Think you're too old for strength training? Think again. Older people—even those in their nineties—who have been sedentary for years have the most to gain from strength training because they have the weakest muscles. Just twelve weeks of strength training has been found to triple muscular strength and increase the number of calories needed to maintain body weight by 15 percent in older people. Many hospital-affiliated wellness centers offer strength-training programs and expert guidance for older people.

STRATEGIES FOR SUCCESS

Many people go on and off their exercise regimens, just as they go on and off their diets. How can you keep your motivation high? First, make exercise fun by incorporating it into your family and social life. Substitute walking, hiking, canoeing, biking, racquet sports, and other healthful activities for sedentary ones, like going to happy hour, watching television, and playing computer games. This way, it won't be just one more thing to do.

Second, start slowly and increase your workouts gradually. Being an overzealous exerciser will likely cause injury, burnout, or both. And take every precaution you can to prevent dehydration and injury. For instance, drink plenty of water before, during, and after exercise, and plan your workouts so that you avoid the hottest part of the day. Always stretch before and after a workout. Just as important, purchase the proper equipment for your sport—good walking shoes or a bike helmet, for instance. If you're not sure about what you're doing, consult an expert. Many community colleges and hospital wellness centers offer adult fitness classes taught by exercise physiologists. Personal trainers are another option, but make sure that your personal trainer is qualified by asking to see his or her certification. Trainers should either have a college degree in exercise physiology, be certified by an agency such as the American College of Sports Medicine (ACSM), or both. Finally, if you are over forty years of age or have specific health problems, be sure to check with your physician before starting any exercise program.

The bottom line is that exercise is an effective and necessary part of any health-promoting lifestyle. It supports weight loss, it relieves stress, and it helps reduce the risk of a variety of health problems. For maximum health benefits, you should be sure to include both aerobic exercise and strength-training activities in your exercise regimen. And you should exercise about thirty minutes a day—enough to burn a minimum of 150 calories. Most important, make exercise fun by incorporating it into your social life. Get friends and family involved, and choose an activity that you will find enjoyable and will look forward to doing each and every day.

Conclusion

If you've gotten this far, you've taken a major step toward achieving a healthier lifestyle. The next step is to take what you've learned and put it into practice. Unfortunately, the simple act of reading this book will not lower your fat intake. Only by incorporating your new-found strategies into your everyday activities will you be able to reap the benefits that others have enjoyed—benefits like greater weight control, increased energy, and reduced risk of heart disease, diabetes, and cancer.

Experience has shown that the tips, guidelines, and strategies presented in this book *do* work. However, they are not the only ways to cut down on fat. Don't be afraid to devise your own secrets of fat-free living. You may come up with great new ways of avoiding the fat traps in restaurants, on the road, or in your own kitchen. Then, if you'd like to share your ideas, please don't hesitate to write to me, care of the publisher. I wish you luck in all your fat-free endeavors.

Metric Conversion Tables

Conversion Table

LIQUID

When You Know	Multiply By	To Determine
teaspoons	5.0	milliliters
tablespoons	15.0	milliliters
fluid ounces	30.0	milliliters
cups	0.24	liters
pints	0.47	liters
quarts	0.95	liters

WEIGHT

When You Know	Multiply By	To Determine
ounces	28.0	grams
pounds	0.45	kilograms

Common Liquid Conversions

Measurement	=	Liters
1/4 cup	=	0.06 liters
1/2 cup	=	0.12 liters
3/4 cup	=	0.18 liters
1 cup	=	0.24 liters
1 1/4 cups	=	0.30 liters
1 1/2 cups	=	0.36 liters
2 cups	=	0.48 liters
2 1/2 cups	=	0.60 liters
3 cups	=	0.72 liters
3 1/2 cups	=	0.84 liters
4 cups	=	0.96 liters
4 1/2 cups	=	1.08 liters
5 cups	=	1.20 liters
5 1/2 cups	=	1.32 liters

Measurement	=	Milliliters
1/4 teaspoon	=	1.25 milliliters
1/2 teaspoon	=	2.50 milliliters
3/4 teaspoon	=	3.75 milliliters
1 teaspoon	=	5.00 milliliters
1 1/4 teaspoons	=	6.25 milliliters
1 1/2 teaspoons	=	7.50 milliliters
1 3/4 teaspoons	=	8.75 milliliters
2 teaspoons	=	10.0 milliliters
1 tablespoon	=	15.0 milliliters
2 tablespoons	=	30.0 milliliters

Converting Fahrenheit to Celsius

Fahrenheit	=	Celsius
200—205	=	95
220—225	=	105
245—250	=	120
275	=	135
300—305	=	150
325—330	=	165
345—350	=	175
370—375	=	190
400—405	=	205
425—430	=	220
445—450	=	230
470—475	=	245
500	=	260

Index

Healthy Habits

are easy to come by—

IF YOU KNOW WHERE TO LOOK!

Get the latest information on:

- better health • diet & weight loss
- the latest nutritional supplements
- herbal healing • homeopathy and more

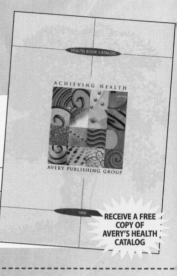

COMPLETE AND RETURN THIS CARD RIGHT AWAY!

Where did you purchase this book?

- ❑ bookstore
- ❑ health food store
- ❑ pharmacy
- ❑ supermarket
- ❑ other (please specify)_____

Name_____

Street Address_____

City_____State____Zip_____

RECEIVE A FREE COPY OF AVERY'S HEALTH CATALOG

GIVE ONE TO A FRIEND ...

Healthy Habits

are easy to come by—

IF YOU KNOW WHERE TO LOOK!

Get the latest information on:

- better health • diet & weight loss
- the latest nutritional supplements
- herbal healing • homeopathy and more

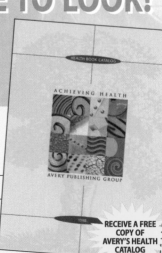

COMPLETE AND RETURN THIS CARD RIGHT AWAY!

Where did you purchase this book?

- ❑ bookstore
- ❑ health food store
- ❑ pharmacy
- ❑ supermarket
- ❑ other (please specify)_____

Name_____

Street Address_____

City_____State____Zip_____

RECEIVE A FREE COPY OF AVERY'S HEALTH CATALOG

Avery Publishing Group

120 Old Broadway
Garden City Park, NY 11040

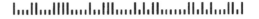

Avery Publishing Group

120 Old Broadway
Garden City Park, NY 11040